Salmonella - Molecular Biology, Pathogenesis, and Public Health Impact

Edited by Mihaela Laura Vica

Published in London, United Kingdom

Salmonella - Molecular Biology, Pathogenesis, and Public Health Impact
http://dx.doi.org/10.5772/intechopen.1009714
Edited by Mihaela Laura Vica

Contributors
Aayushi Patel, Adedeji O. Adetunji, Adioumani A. Emmanuella, Adishi Ranjan, Ainyakou-Sanga Aiza Monique, Ana R. Miljković, Andrew Wolfram, Barro Nicolas, Derrick A. Daah, E.M. Nikiema Marguerite, Emmanuel Asiamah, Goualie Gblossi Bernadette, Greeshma Bharathan, Heidi Price, Henrietta Owusu, Imad Mohamedtahir Fadlalla, Kakou-Ngazoa E. Solange, Karou Germain, Kipre Christ Romuald, Margery Claude-Charlène Keke, Melis Gönülal, Obou Constantin Okou, Olumuyiwa Olarotimi, Ouattara Zeinab, Samuel Duodu, Seetha Lakshmi, Shabarinath Srikumar, Taseen S. Desin, Thomas P. Oscar

First published in London, United Kingdom, 2026 by IntechOpen
IntechOpen is the global imprint of INTECHOPEN LIMITED, registered in England and Wales, registration number: 11086078, 167-169 Great Portland Street, London, W1W 5PF, United Kingdom

For EU product safety concerns: IN TECH d.o.o., Prolaz Marije Krucifikse Kozulić 3, 51000 Rijeka, Croatia, info@intechopen.com or visit our website at intechopen.com.

British Library Cataloguing-in-Publication Data
A catalogue record for this book is available from the British Library

Salmonella - Molecular Biology, Pathogenesis, and Public Health Impact
Edited by Mihaela Laura Vica
p. cm.
Print ISBN 978-1-83635-629-5
Online ISBN 978-1-83635-628-8
eBook (PDF) ISBN 978-1-83635-630-1

If disposing of this product, please recycle the paper responsibly.

Meet the editor

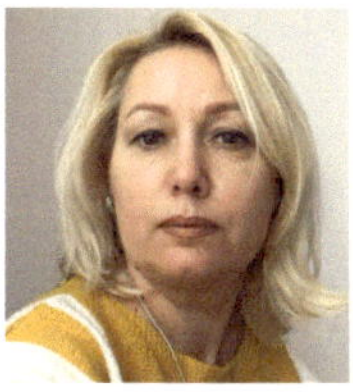

Dr. Mihaela Laura Vică, MSc, Ph.D., is an Associate Professor in the Department of Cell and Molecular Biology at the "Iuliu Hațieganu" University of Medicine and Pharmacy, Romania, where she obtained her Ph.D. in Medicine. She obtained her MSc in Cellular Biology from the Faculty of Biology, "Babeş-Bolyai" University, Romania. Since 2006, Dr. Vică has been involved in scientific research, coordinating an international cooperation research project and participating in over 40 national and international conferences, during which she has received 5 awards. She has published one book as editor, two books as co-author, three book chapters, and more than eighty research papers in extenso in international journals. Her areas of research are microbiology and molecular biology.

Contents

Preface

Salmonella is a Gram-negative bacterium, a member of the *Enterobacteriaceae*, that causes infections in both animals and humans. *Salmonella* has been identified as an important food and water-borne pathogen that can infect organisms, resulting in significant morbidity and mortality. Besides its known role in food poisoning, this bacterium has long been recognized as one of the most common causes of systemic infections. For this reason, significant efforts have been made to prevent its spread, but *Salmonella* infection nevertheless remains a major public health problem in both developed and developing countries. With the emergence of multidrug-resistant strains in recent years, treating *Salmonella* infections has become increasingly challenging.

Salmonella – Molecular Biology, Pathogenesis, and Public Health Impact provides current information on various aspects of *Salmonella* infections, from contamination risks and bacterial spread to treatment, prevention, and control. The chapters are authored by recognized experts in the field, who provide valuable information about *Salmonella* infections, drawing on both their own experience and the existing literature.

Various aspects related to this bacterium are discussed, such as molecular structures and mechanisms, new therapeutic approaches, the importance of modern detection techniques, the genetic mechanisms of antibiotic resistance, and the transmission of resistance genes. Additionally, topics such as contamination risk assessment and future strategies to prevent the spread of this bacterium are also addressed.

Since *Salmonella* infections are a major cause of death in many parts of the world, particularly in developing countries, the first three chapters of this book focus on the public health impact of *Salmonella* in different regions worldwide. The first two chapters provide information about salmonellosis in Africa, focusing on its burden, biology, evolution, pathogenesis, antimicrobial resistance, and diagnostic and surveillance capabilities available in these regions. Chapter 3 provides an overview of contemporary epidemiological trends in Europe, examining regional differences, seasonal patterns, and the most common sources of infection.

The following three chapters detail aspects of the mechanisms involved in transmission, dissemination of disease, virulence, or antimicrobial resistance in *Salmonella*. Understanding the mechanisms behind drug resistance and its transmission is essential for improved monitoring and control. One of the chapters provides a comprehensive analysis of the role of poultry matrices in the transmission dynamics of *Salmonella*, including the pathogen's biology, virulence mechanisms, and environmental adaptability. Chapter 5 explores the molecular basis of Non-typhoidal *Salmonella* (NTS) pathogenesis, reviews emerging multidrug-resistant strains, and discusses current strategies for controlling transmission. Chapter 6 examines the mechanisms by which *Salmonella* causes disease in livestock, emphasizing the dynamics of host-pathogen interactions that contribute to intestinal inflammation and septicemia. It also explores the role of antibiotics in mitigating salmonellosis.

The next two chapters in this book address *Salmonella* diseases. One chapter focuses on skin adverse reactions caused by *Salmonella* infections, which, although rare, can be severe and often difficult to identify as the causative factor. The other chapter in this section addresses *Salmonella* infections and evaluates the antibacterial activity of a food plant as an alternative therapy due to increasing resistance to standard antibiotic treatments.

The book ends with two theoretical chapters on risk analysis and future approaches. Chapter 9 analyzes computer models that predict consumer exposure and response to *Salmonella* in poultry food, while the final chapter highlights the importance of the One Health Approach in *Salmonella* public health, particularly in obtaining a comprehensive picture of bacterial antimicrobial resistance.

I would like to thank all the authors for their contributions and the time spent preparing this valuable collection. I would also like to extend my thanks to the staff at IntechOpen, particularly Ms. Tea Jelaca, for their invaluable help during the editing of this book.

Mihaela Laura Vică, MSc, Ph.D.
Cell and Molecular Biology Department,
"Iuliu Hațieganu" University of Medicine and Pharmacy,
Cluj-Napoca, Romania

Section 1

Public Health Impact of *Salmonella*

Chapter 1

Circulating of *Salmonella* Strains in West Africa: Lacks of Surveillance and Research

Kakou-Ngazoa Evelyne Solange,
Nikiema Marguerite Edith Malatala,
Goualie Gblossi Bernadette, Ainyakou-Sanga Aiza Monique,
Kipré Christ Romuald, Ouattara Zeinab,
Adioumani A. Emmanuella, Barro Nicolas and Karou Germain

Abstract

Salmonella is one of the main causes of diarrheal infections worldwide, particularly in tropical and subtropical regions. In West Africa, several *Salmonella* strains have been identified and characterised, revealing an alarming trend towards the emergence and spread of multidrug-resistant (MDR) strains. Despite this serious situation, epidemiological surveillance remains limited and insufficient on a national scale. The main transmission routes, particularly foodborne transmission, as well as inadequate hygiene and health-and-safety practices, play a significant role in the dissemination of these resistant strains within the region. This study aims to provide an up-to-date overview of salmonellosis in West Africa, focusing on antimicrobial resistance dynamics and the diagnostic and surveillance capabilities available. It also proposes alternative therapeutic and control strategies. This analysis is in line with the One Health approach, which is advocated as an integrative framework for multisectoral surveillance of antimicrobial resistance in tropical contexts, and for rationalising antibiotic use in human, animal and environmental health.

Keywords: *Salmonella*, detection, West Africa, MDR, one health, phage therapy

1. Introduction

Salmonellosis, which is caused by typhoidal and non-typhoidal strains of *Salmonella enterica*, poses a significant threat to public health in West Africa. Non-typhoidal strains (NTS) are of particular concern, as they cause a variety of clinical syndromes, including gastroenteritis, septicaemia and invasive systemic infections, particularly in children, immunocompromised individuals, malnourished individuals and patients with malaria [1]. In tropical regions, the high prevalence of these risk factors makes populations particularly vulnerable to these severe infections.

Several studies conducted in Burkina Faso between 2008 and 2020 have documented the circulation of *Salmonella* in various samples. A summary of these data indicates an average prevalence of 4.6% in humans, 20.1% in animals, 16.8% in food and 15.6% in the environment [2]. A recent systematic review and meta-analysis by Traore et al. [2] have confirmed these data and highlights the widespread presence of non-typhoidal strains in all human, animal, food and environmental compartments in Burkina Faso. The study reports high diversity among the circulating serotypes, which are associated with virulence and resistance genes. This indicates significant pathogenic and epidemic potential [2].

The situation is also alarming in other countries in the subregion. In Côte d'Ivoire, for example, a study of ready-to-eat foods, particularly street salads, found that 8.5% were contaminated with *Salmonella*. The study also found nalidixic acid and ciprofloxacin resistance, as well as resistance genes such as *tetA, tetB* and *qnrA* [3]. In Ghana, *Salmonella* strains have been isolated from dust, soil, water, poultry and human patients. The most frequently identified serotypes include *S*. Typhimurium, *S*. Enteritidis and *S*. Kentucky, which are all known to be involved in invasive forms of the disease and to frequently exhibit antibiotic resistance [4]. A systematic review conducted in Niger by Abdelkader et al. [5] based on 25 relevant publications showed that the dominant serotypes in humans in Africa are *S*. Typhimurium, *S*. Enteritidis and *S*. Typhi, while *S*. Hadar dominates in poultry, except in North Africa, where *S*. Typhimurium is more prevalent [5].

A meta-analysis of avian strains collected in Africa between 2000 and 2020 reports an average prevalence of 14.4% in poultry, with 141 serotypes identified in West Africa. The most common serotypes are *S*. Enteritidis, *S*. Typhimurium, *S*. Kentucky and *S*. Hadar [6]. Additionally, invasive non-typical strains (iNTS), particularly the ST313 (*S*. Typhimurium) and ST11 (*S*. Enteritidis) genomic lineages, have been linked to severe haematogenous infections in various countries within the region. Without appropriate treatment, these infections often prove fatal, with estimated case fatality rates of 15–25% [7].

Nikiema et al. [8, 9] conducted a study of fast food (sandwiches) sold on the streets of Ouagadougou, highlighting a particularly worrying finding. Of the 201 samples analysed, 17.9% were contaminated with *S. enterica*, representing 16 different serotypes, including *S*. Kentucky, *S*. Derby and *S*. Tennessee [8]. Multiresistant clones were identified, including the ST198-X1 clone of *S*. Kentucky, which is known for spreading internationally, as well as an invasive lineage of *S*. Enteritidis belonging to the West African clade. Several isolates were found to have virulence genes such as *invA, stn, fimA, spvR* and *spvC*, which supports the idea that the street food preparation and sales chain is a significant route of transmission to humans [9]. Similarly, Somda et al. [10] demonstrated the presence of these virulence genes in strains isolated in Burkina Faso, confirming their critical role in the pathogenicity and spread of local strains [10]. In addition, Deguenon et al. [11] reported an association between virulence genes and antibiotic resistance in *Salmonella* strains isolated from slaughtered animals in Benin. This suggests a significant zoonotic risk associated with consuming meat products [11]. This issue is particularly critical given that more than 80% of the population consume informal urban meals daily, in a context marked by inadequate sanitary infrastructure and a lack of microbiological food control. The risk of the collective spread of pathogenic and multiresistant strains is therefore extremely high.

2. Antimicrobial resistance (AMR) in *Salmonella* in West Africa

Antimicrobial resistance (AMR) in *Salmonella* enterica poses a significant health challenge in West Africa. This issue is exacerbated by the uncontrolled and frequently inappropriate use of antibiotics in human and veterinary medicine and agricultural practices. A lack of strict regulatory policies, coupled with widespread self-medication and prophylactic antimicrobial use in livestock farming, promotes the emergence and dissemination of multidrug-resistant (MDR) strains [12]. Cross-sectional studies conducted in several countries in the region have highlighted the presence of resistant strains in hospitals, livestock farms, food markets and urban environments [2]. A recent meta-analysis of non-typhoidal *Salmonella* (NTS) in sub-Saharan Africa revealed high rates of resistance to ampicillin (66%), trimethoprim-sulfamethoxazole (33%) and chloramphenicol (28%) [2]. In Burkina Faso, recent studies have confirmed the emergence and circulation of resistant clones in the human, animal, food and environmental sectors. Nikiema et al. [8] found that over 50% of *Salmonella* isolates from street sandwiches and patients' stools with diarrhoea were multidrug-resistant. Frequent resistance was observed to ampicillin, tetracycline, streptomycin, nalidixic acid and ciprofloxacin [8]. Notably, the epidemic clone *S.* Kentucky ST198-X1, carrying mutations in *gyrA* and *parC* that confer high resistance to fluoroquinolones, was identified. This highlights the potential for highly pathogenic and difficult-to-treat strains to spread [8, 13].

In the poultry sector, Kagambèga et al. [14] revealed alarming levels of antibiotic resistance in strains isolated from chicken carcasses, droppings, drinking troughs and slaughtering surfaces in Ouagadougou. These strains exhibited high levels of resistance to tetracycline (93.8%), ampicillin (68.8%) and chloramphenicol (59.4%). The presence of resistance genes, such as *tet(A), sul1,* $bla_{\text{TEM-1B}}$, and *aadA1*, suggests intense antibiotic pressure in urban farming systems [14]. The convergence of food, environmental and clinical sources underscores the pivotal role of the food chain in AMR dynamics. Street food, which is widespread in urban areas, thus appears to be a critical link in this chain. A complementary study by Nikiema et al. [9] showed that *Salmonella* isolates present in sandwiches co-occurred with resistance and virulence genes, indicating an increased risk to public health.

Similar data have been reported in several neighbouring countries beyond Burkina Faso. For example, a study conducted in Niger in 2015 among children with diarrhoea revealed the circulation of several *Salmonella* serotypes, primarily *S.* Typhimurium (20%), *S.* Enteritidis (15.8%) and *S.* Corvallis (13%) [15]. Around 13% of the isolates exhibited an ESBL phenotype, and over half of the enterobacteria were resistant to amoxicillin and cotrimoxazole. In a context of persistent child malnutrition, these infections increase the risk of severe forms, even if they are not directly responsible for diarrhoea. In Ghana, Nigeria, Benin and Senegal, fluoroquinolone and third-generation cephalosporin-resistant strains have been isolated, some of which carry $bla_{\text{TEM-1B}}$, $bla_{\text{CTX-M}}$, bla_{OXA} or qnr genes [16]. These profiles are characteristic of strains with a high risk of epidemic spread, which are often associated with mobile genetic elements such as conjugative plasmids.

In the face of this critical situation, the World Health Organisation (WHO) recommends adopting a 'One Health' approach, which considers the human, animal and environmental aspects together in order to combat AMR. The aim is to strengthen integrated surveillance systems, such as the Global Antimicrobial Resistance Surveillance System (GLASS), and improve diagnostic capabilities, including molecular microbiology and sequencing. The approach also seeks to promote the prudent use of antimicrobials in all sectors and develop alternatives to antibiotics in animal production chains

[17]. However, effective implementation of this approach in this region is hindered by several challenges, including a lack of intersectoral coordination, inadequate laboratory infrastructure, and an absence of coherent national monitoring and control programmes. Prioritising the development of local capacity, particularly in the fields of microbiology and genomics, is essential to halting the spread of AMR in the region.

3. Detection capacity of *Salmonella* in West Africa

Studies on *Salmonella* in West Africa generally focus on strains originating from food (meat, milk, eggs, street food, vegetables, etc.), animals (poultry, fish, pigs, etc.), water, humans (faeces and blood) and environmental samples. The isolation and identification of *Salmonella* in West Africa rely largely on conventional methods standardised by the WHO, ISO, and, in some cases, the internal protocols of national laboratories. However, local constraints, such as technical and financial resources, often influence the choice of methods used.

3.1 Standard techniques in West Africa for the isolation and identification of *Salmonella*

In general, the isolation method used is based on ISO 6579-2005 for the analysis of food, as well as samples of animal and environmental origin.

The analyses are conducted in three main steps. First, pre-enrichment of 25 g of the sample in 225 ml of Buffered Peptone Water (BPW) or trypticase soy broth during 24 h at 37°C followed by an enrichment using a selective medium, which may be either Rappaport-Vassiliadis (RV) broth [8, 18–20], Tetrathionate (TT) broth, or Selenite Cystine medium [21] at 37–42°C for 6–24 h. Finally, isolation is performed on a selective agar medium by the streak plate method. The most commonly used culture media are Xylose Lysine Deoxycholate (XLD) agar, Hektoen Enteric agar, Salmonella-Shigella (SS) agar and MacConkey (MAC) agar [22]. Other agar media, such as Brilliant Green agar, are also reported.

In some studies, isolation is carried out in two steps, both from human samples (blood and faeces) and from animal-derived samples. In these protocols, enrichment is performed directly in Selenite broth or brain-heart infusion broth at 37°C for 18–24 h followed by isolation on Salmonella-Shigella agar at 37°C for 24 h [8, 18–21, 23, 24].

Identification of *Salmonella* strains in most studies is based on morphological (macroscopic and microscopic), biochemical, and molecular characteristics. Biochemical identification is generally performed using the reduced Le Minor test kit or the API 20E system. In some studies, standard techniques as described by Cowan and Steel [25] and Cruickshank et al. [26] are used for biochemical identification [23].

Molecular identification targets specific virulence genes of the *Salmonella* genus, notably the *invA* gene [18, 20], *fimA, stn, spvC* or the *spvR* genes [9, 11]. However, these biochemical and molecular methods are limited to identifying the genus *Salmonella* and do not allow determination of the specific serotype.

3.2 *Salmonella* serotyping methods in the west African laboratories

Salmonella serotyping plays a central role in the identification of this genus. It enables differentiation of strains within the species and links laboratory findings to epidemiological surveillance by mapping the geographical distribution of strains [27].

The most widely used reference method in studies reported in West Africa is serotyping according to the White-Kauffmann-Le Minor (WKLM) scheme. This method is based on the identification of O (somatic) and H (flagellar, phases 1 and 2) antigens, as well as the capsular Vi antigen (particularly in certain serovars), using slide agglutination tests [6]. However, In the West African context, where laboratory resources and infrastructure are often limited, the WKLM scheme remains the gold standard for comprehensive *Salmonella* serotyping but is constrained by high costs, reagent availability, and the need for highly trained personnel [28].

A study conducted on *Salmonella* strains isolated from human, initially in Ghana and subsequently in other West African countries, including Burkina Faso, Guinee-Bissau and Senegal, tested and validated a rapid molecular typing method in comparison with the traditional WKLM serotyping scheme [29]. In this study, the authors applied both the classical serotyping method and a multiplex PCR targeting major serovars, namely *S.* Typhi, *S.* Typhimurium, *S.* Dublin and *S.* Enteritidis [29]. Multiplex PCR offers a rapid, cost-effective and less labour-intensive alternative for the detection of priority serovars, enabling faster decision-making in outbreak investigations and routine surveillance. However, its coverage is limited to the serovars included in the assay design, meaning it cannot fully replace the WKLM method. A combined approach using multiplex PCR for rapid initial screening and WKLM serotyping for confirmatory analysis and epidemiological reporting could therefore provide an efficient, context-appropriate strategy to strengthen *Salmonella* surveillance and control efforts in the region [29].

3.3 Techniques for assessing antibiotic resistance

Antibiotic resistance has become one of the major public health concerns worldwide. Consequently, the determination of antibiotic resistance profiles is routinely performed in most laboratories in West Africa. The most commonly applied method is the Kirby-Bauer disc diffusion technique on Mueller-Hinton agar, as recommended by the CASFM/EUCAST, alongside the determination of minimum inhibitory concentrations (MICs) according to the guidelines of the Clinical and Laboratory Standards Institute (CLSI) [14, 24, 30, 31]. Typically, between nine (9) [32] and twenty-two (22) antimicrobial agents may be tested, with the interpretation of results based on CASFM/EUCAST guidelines [18, 20, 24, 33] or CLSI recommendations [4, 24, 30]. These methods have consistently revealed an alarming increase in *Salmonella* resistance rates to various antibiotics, as well as the emergence of cross-resistance and multidrug resistance (MDR) profiles [34]. Many studies have also focused on the genetic determinants of resistance [30, 35] using molecular biology techniques such as PCR and sequencing to detect specific mutations within target genes. The most frequently identified resistance genes are those conferring resistance to β-lactams (e.g., (bla_{TEM}, bla_{CTX}, bla_{SHV} and AmpC) [30, 35, 36], to fluoroquinolones (due to chromosomal mutations in *gyrA* and *parC* genes, as well as plasmid-mediated *qnrA, qnrB, qnrS*) [35, 37–41], to tetracyclines (*tetA, tetB*), to sulphonamides (sul1, sul2), and to trimethoprim (various *dfr* genes such as *dfrA1, dfrA12*) [30].

3.4 Genotyping techniques for *Salmonella* in West Africa

Some studies conducted in West Africa focusing on the use of various genotyping methods have been reported. These various methods enable fine differentiation of strains, thereby allowing the tracing of contamination chains and improving epidemiological surveillance of *Salmonella* infections.

Indeed, research conducted by Al-Emran et al. [29] validated a multiplex PCR technique for the rapid identification of common serovars (e.g., *Salmonella* Typhi, Typhimurium, Dublin, Enteritidis), based on the detection of genes corresponding to O and H antigens. This technique, regularly applied in Ghana and Burkina Faso for typhoid fever surveillance, remains rapid, relatively inexpensive and well-suited to laboratories in the region where PCR equipment is still of a standard type [29, 42].

Other studies in Nigeria [39, 43, 44] have demonstrated the potential to explore clonal relationships among strains isolated from humans, animals and the environment through next-generation sequencing (NGS) for whole-genome sequencing (WGS) of each isolate. These authors highlighted the high potential of applied genomic tools—particularly NGS—in tracing the origin and epidemiological links of outbreak strains.

In Burkina Faso, WGS using NGS coupled with multilocus sequence typing (MLST) has been performed to analyse *Salmonella enterica* serovar Enteritidis and *Salmonella enterica* serovar Typhimurium strains originating from poultry and humans [8, 14, 45]. The authors identified resistance genes and chromosomal mutations specific to the strains studied, as well as mobile genetic elements (e.g., plasmids, transposons), suggesting the potential for horizontal gene transfer and, consequently, environmental dissemination. Moreover, they demonstrated that isolates from poultry and humans were genetically closely related, representing a potential food safety risk to consumers [14]. The application of NGS in another Nigerian study led to the creation of a draft genome sequence database from 37 *Salmonella enterica* strains of avian origin. According to the authors, these data were deposited in public data banks (GenBank, DDBJ, EMBL) and can serve as references for improving *Salmonella* traceability studies as well as foodborne disease surveillance [46].

In Sierra Leone, real-time PCR and NGS were applied to the samples from patients with fever in Freetown with the aim of improving the reliability of typhoid fever and invasive salmonellosis diagnoses, and especially to replace unreliable traditional methods (e.g., the Widal test) with modern molecular techniques such as quantitative PCR (qPCR) and next-generation sequencing (NGS) [47].

In summary, in West Africa, PCR methods are commonly used for rapid typing, while WGS is gaining ground due to its analytical power. The use of these techniques provides key genomic data on various characteristics of *Salmonella* strains from diverse origins, notably the factors responsible for antibiotic resistance and their virulence aptitudes, the circulating serotypes, and, most importantly, the existence of clonal links between animal, environmental and human strains within a One Health context. However, these techniques remain largely inaccessible to most laboratories in this African region.

4. Strategies for *Salmonella* research in West Africa

For an effective *Salmonella* research strategy in West Africa, the following actions are essential:

- Establish strong collaborations among laboratories across West African countries to promote the pooling of equipment and resources, thereby enabling less well-equipped laboratories to implement modern techniques for studying this bacterial genus, including PCR, next-generation sequencing (NGS) and multilocus sequence typing (MLST).

- Form multidisciplinary and cross-sectoral research teams to ensure integrated surveillance of this pathogen across the subregion.
- Create a multi-country sentinel network for efficient monitoring of circulating serovars.
- Develop a West African biobank and a centralised database compiling whole-genome sequencing (WGS) data on isolates from diverse origins. These initiatives should help address key research questions, such as:
- Which serovars or clones are predominant in each country and along specific production chains?
- Which genes and plasmids are most frequently associated with antimicrobial resistance (AMR) in West Africa, and what strategies are currently employed in each country for AMR surveillance?
- What are the highest-risk behaviours and the most critical control points identified within the transmission chain?
- What is the true prevalence of *Salmonella* infections in each country of the subregion?

Ultimately, the implementation of a robust *Salmonella* research strategy should focus on reducing the burden of both non-typhoidal and typhoidal *Salmonella* infections through a One Health approach in West Africa. This approach would integrate surveillance, genomics, risk assessment and field interventions across the entire food chain (pork, poultry, beef, fish, high-risk vegetables, street food, restaurant-prepared meals), while considering the human-animal-environment interface.

5. Phage therapy for *Salmonella* in Africa

Foodborne microbial diseases continue to be a serious food safety problem worldwide. In addition to their public health significance, the economic impact of foodborne bacterial infections is considerable. Preventing contamination and providing a safe food supply are the two high-priority areas for controlling and limiting foodborne pathogen outbreaks within the One Health approach [48]. Currently, conventional pathogen decontamination protocols are used in food processing facilities.

In Africa, Egypt has confirmed the efficacy of phages against multiresistant strains of *Salmonella* in ready-to-eat foods and in broiler chicken [49, 50]. Worldwide, many studies report the uses of phages for One Health purposes (Food products/veterinary medicine). This suggests that these phages could play a dual role: not only effectively reducing zoonotic *Salmonella* strains, thus lowering FBO risk, but also limiting the transmission of AMR *Salmonella* to humans [51].

6. Conclusion

For phage therapy to effectively complement strategies to combat antibiotic resistance, several actions need to be considered:

1. Local capacity building: Investing in training researchers and healthcare professionals on phage isolation, characterisation and use is crucial. Partnerships with international institutions could facilitate knowledge and technology transfer between Phagenetworks and the Food industries, Academic institutions.

2. Infrastructure development: The creation of laboratories with phage production capacities, as well as the establishment of phage banks.

3. Regulatory framework: Health authorities must develop clear guidelines for the approval and use of phages, drawing on successful experiences in other regions of the world.

4. Awareness and acceptance: Information campaigns targeting healthcare professionals and the general public are essential to promote phage therapy and allay fears related to its use.

5. One Health approach in agriculture, and animal production must be urgently considered phages uses for reduction of antibiotics uses in Africa.

Author details

Kakou-Ngazoa Evelyne Solange[1*], Nikiema Marguerite Edith Malatala[2,3], Goualie Gblossi Bernadette[4], Ainyakou-Sanga Aiza Monique[4], Kipré Christ Romuald[4], Ouattara Zeinab[1], Adioumani A. Emmanuella[1], Barro Nicolas[3] and Karou Germain[4]

1 Pasteur Institute Cote d'Ivoire, Platform of Molecular Biology, Abidjan, Côte d'Ivoire

2 Laboratoire de Virologie et de Biotechnologies Végétales, Institut de l'Environnement et de Recherches Agricoles (LVBV/INERA), Centre National de la Recherche Scientifique et Technologique (CNRST), Ouagadougou, Burkina Faso

3 Laboratoire de Biologie moléculaire, d'Epidémiologie et de Surveillance des agents Transmissibles par les Aliments (LaBESTA), Ecole Doctorale Sciences et Technologies, Université Joseph KI- ZERBO, Ouagadougou, Burkina Faso

4 Department of Biotechnology, Unit of Training and Research in Biosciences, Félix HOUPHOUËT-BOIGNY University, Abidjan, Côte d'Ivoire

*Address all correspondence to: ngazoa_solange@yahoo.fr and solangekakou@pasteur.ci

References

[1] Ao TT, Feasey NA, Gordon MA, Keddy KH, Angulo FJ, Crump JA. Global burden of invasive nontyphoidal Salmonella disease, 2010(1). Emerging Infectious Diseases. 2015;**21**:941-949. DOI: 10.3201/eid2106.140999

[2] Traore KA, Aboubacar-Paraiso AR, Bouda SC, Ouoba JB, Kagambèga A, Roques P, et al. Characteristics of nontyphoid Salmonella isolated from human, environmental, animal, and food samples in Burkina Faso: A systematic review and meta-analysis. Antibiotics. 2024;**13**:556. DOI: 10.3390/antibiotics13060556

[3] Toe E, Attien P, Moroh AJ-L, Sina H, Kouame DN, Kambire O, et al. Prevalence and characterization of Salmonella isolated from vegetables salads and ready to eat raw mixed vegetable salads in Abidjan, Cte dIvoire. Journal of Microbiology and Antimicrobials. 2022;**14**:15-25. DOI: 10.5897/JMA2021.0449

[4] Andoh LA, Ahmed S, Olsen JE, Obiri-Danso K, Newman MJ, Opintan JA, et al. Prevalence and characterization of Salmonella among humans in Ghana. Tropical Medicine and Health. 2017;**45**:3. DOI: 10.1186/s41182-017-0043-z

[5] Abdelkader AS, Oumarou SS, Maârouhi IM, Ali DB, Yacoubou B. Prévalence Et Diversité De Salmonella En Afrique: Analyse Qualitative Et Quantitative. European Scientific Journal. 2017;**13**:250-250. DOI: 10.19044/esj.2017.v13n30p250

[6] Kabeta T, Tolosa T, Duchateau L, Van Immerseel F, Antonissen G. Prevalence and serotype of poultry salmonellosis in Africa: A systematic review and meta-analysis. Avian Pathology. 2024;**53**:325-349. DOI: 10.1080/03079457.2024.2344549

[7] Feasey NA, Dougan G, Kingsley RA, Heyderman RS, Gordon MA. Invasive non-typhoidal Salmonella disease: An emerging and neglected tropical disease in Africa. Lancet. 2012;**379**:2489-2499. DOI: 10.1016/S0140-6736(11)61752-2

[8] Nikiema MEM, de la Gandara MP, Compaore KAM, Ba AK, Soro KD, Nikiema PA, et al. Contamination of street food with multidrug-resistant Salmonella, in Ouagadougou, Burkina Faso. PLoS One. 2021a;**16**:e0253312. DOI: 10.1371/journal.pone.0253312

[9] Nikiema MEM, Kakou-Ngazoa S, Ky/Ba A, Sylla A, Bako E, Addablah AYA, et al. Characterization of virulence factors of Salmonella isolated from human stools and street food in urban areas of Burkina Faso. BMC Microbiology. 2021b;**21**:338. DOI: 10.1186/s12866-021-02398-6

[10] Somda NS, Bonkoungou IJO, Sambe-Ba B, Drabo MS, Wane AA, Sawadogo-Lingani H, et al. Diversity and antimicrobial drug resistance of non-typhoid *Salmonella* serotypes isolated in lettuce, irrigation water and clinical samples in Burkina Faso. Journal of Agriculture and Food Research. 2021;**5**:100167. DOI: 10.1016/j.jafr.2021.100167

[11] Deguenon E, Dougnon V, Lozes E, Maman N, Agbankpe J, Abdel-Massih RM, et al. Resistance and virulence determinants of faecal Salmonella spp. isolated from slaughter animals in Benin. BMC Research Notes. 2019;**12**:317. DOI: 10.1186/s13104-019-4341-x

[12] Van Boeckel TP, Brower C, Gilbert M, Grenfell BT, Levin SA, Robinson TP, et al. Global trends in antimicrobial use in food animals. Proceedings of the National Academy of Sciences of the United States of America. 2015;**112**:5649-5654. DOI: 10.1073/pnas.1503141112

[13] Le Hello S, Hendriksen RS, Doublet B, Fisher I, Nielsen EM, Whichard JM, et al. International spread of an epidemic population of *Salmonella enterica* serotype Kentucky ST198 resistant to ciprofloxacin. The Journal of Infectious Diseases. 2011;**204**:675-684. DOI: 10.1093/infdis/jir409

[14] Kagambèga A, Lienemann T, Frye JG, Barro N, Haukka K. Whole genome sequencing of multidrug-resistant *Salmonella enterica* serovar Typhimurium isolated from humans and poultry in Burkina Faso. Tropical Medicine and Health. 2018;**46**:4. DOI: 10.1186/s41182-018-0086-9

[15] Langendorf C, Le Hello S, Moumouni A, Gouali M, Mamaty A-A, Grais RF, et al. Enteric bacterial pathogens in children with diarrhea in Niger: Diversity and antimicrobial resistance. PLoS One. 2015;**10**:e0120275. DOI: 10.1371/journal.pone.0120275

[16] Tadesse G, Tessema TS, Beyene G, Aseffa A. Molecular epidemiology of fluoroquinolone resistant Salmonella in Africa: A systematic review and meta-analysis. PLoS One. 2018;**13**:e0192575. DOI: 10.1371/journal.pone.0192575

[17] World Health Organization. Global Antimicrobial Resistance and use Surveillance System (GLASS) Report: 2022 [WWW Document]. 2022. Available from: https://www.who.int/publications/i/item/9789240062702 [Accessed: August 18, 2025]

[18] Ainyakou-Sanga MA, Goualie BG, Kipre RC, Kra DK, Karou GT. Risks associated with the discharge of poultry slaughterhouse waste in public landfill sites in Abidjan, Côte d'Ivoire. Journal of Infection in Developing Countries. 2025;**19**:280-288. DOI: 10.3855/jidc.20125

[19] Bada-Alambedji R, Fofana A, Seydi M, Akakpo AJ. Antimicrobial resistance of Salmonella isolated from poultry carcasses in Dakar (Senegal). Brazilian Journal of Microbiology. 2006;**37**:510-515. DOI: 10.1590/S1517-83822006000400020

[20] Kipré RC, Ainyakou-Sanga MA, Goualie BG, Sylla A, Kra DK, Kakou-NGazoa S, et al. Antimicrobial resistance in Salmonella spp. isolated from poultry waste in Abidjan District, Côte d'ivoire. International Journal of Agriculture and Biosciences. 2025;**14**:643-647. DOI: 10.47278/journal.ijab/2025.036

[21] Ajayi A, Smith SI, Kalpy JC, Bode-Sojobi IO, René YK, Adeleye AI. Molecular diversity and antibiotic resistance gene profile of *Salmonella enterica* serovars isolated from humans and food animals in Lagos, Nigeria. Acta Microbiologica et Immunologica Hungarica. 2019;**66**:509-527. DOI: 10.1556/030.66.2019.034

[22] Dione MM, Ikumapayi U, Saha D, Mohammed NI, Adegbola RA, Geerts S, et al. Antimicrobial resistance and virulence genes of non-typhoidal Salmonella isolates in the Gambia and Senegal. Journal of Infection in Developing Countries. 2011;**5**:765-775. DOI: 10.3855/jidc.1512

[23] Fashae K, Ogunsola F, Aarestrup FM, Hendriksen RS. Antimicrobial susceptibility and serovars of Salmonella from chickens and humans in Ibadan, Nigeria. Journal of Infection in Developing Countries. 2010;**4**:484-494. DOI: 10.3855/jidc.909

[24] Kagambèga A, Lienemann T, Aulu L, Traoré AS, Barro N, Siitonen A, et al. Prevalence and characterization of *Salmonella enterica* from the feces of cattle, poultry, swine and hedgehogs in Burkina Faso and their comparison to human Salmonella isolates. BMC Microbiology. 2013;**13**:253. DOI: 10.1186/1471-2180-13-253

[25] Cowan ST, Steel JP. Manual for the Identification of Medical Bacteria. Cambridge, UK: Cambridge University Press; 1974. pp. 28-106

[26] Cruickshank R, Duguid JP, Marmion BP. Medical Microbiology: The Practice of Medical Microbiology. Edinburgh, UK: Edinburgh Churchill Livingstone; 1975

[27] Tindall BJ, Grimont PAD, Garrity GM, Euzéby JP. Nomenclature and taxonomy of the genus Salmonella. International Journal of Systematic and Evolutionary Microbiology. 2005;**55**:521-524. DOI: 10.1099/ijs.0.63580-0

[28] Wattiau P, Boland C, Bertrand S. Methodologies for *Salmonella enterica* subsp. enterica subtyping: Gold standards and alternatives. Applied and Environmental Microbiology. 2011;**77**:7877-7885. DOI: 10.1128/AEM.05527-11

[29] Al-Emran HM, Krumkamp R, Dekker DM, Eibach D, Aaby P, Adu-Sarkodie Y, et al. Validation and identification of invasive Salmonella serotypes in sub-Saharan Africa by multiplex polymerase chain reaction. Clinical Infectious Diseases. 2016;**62**(Suppl 1):S80-S82. DOI: 10.1093/cid/civ782

[30] Igbinosa EO, Beshiru A, Igbinosa IH, Okoh AI. Antimicrobial resistance and genetic characterisation of *Salmonella enterica* from retail poultry meats in Benin City, Nigeria. LWT. 2022;**169**:114049. DOI: 10.1016/j.lwt.2022.114049

[31] International Typhoid Consortium, Wong VK, Holt KE, Okoro C, Baker S, Pickard DJ, et al. Molecular surveillance identifies multiple transmissions of typhoid in West Africa. PLoS Neglected Tropical Diseases. 2016;**10**:e0004781. DOI: 10.1371/journal.pntd.0004781

[32] Labi A-K, Obeng-Nkrumah N, Addison NO, Donkor ES. Salmonella blood stream infections in a tertiary care setting in Ghana. BMC Infectious Diseases. 2014;**14**:3857. DOI: 10.1186/s12879-014-0697-7

[33] Ofori LA, Fosu D, Ofori S, Akenten CW, Flieger A, Simon S, et al. *Salmonella enterica* in farm environments in the Ashanti region of Ghana. BMC Microbiology. 2023;**23**:370. DOI: 10.1186/s12866-023-03121-3

[34] Assoumy MA, Bedekelabou AP, Teko-Agbo A, Ossebi W, Akoda K, Nimbona F, et al. Antibiotic resistance of Escherichia coli and Salmonella spp. strains isolated from healthy poultry farms in the districts of Abidjan and Agnibilékrou (Côte d'Ivoire). Veterinary World. 2021;**14**:1020-1027. DOI: 10.14202/vetworld.2021.1020-1027

[35] Touglo K, Djeri B, Sina H, Boya B, Ayadokoun GG, Baba-Moussa L, et al. First detection of resistance genes and virulence factors in Escherichia coli and Salmonella spp in Togo: The case of imported chicken and frozen by-products. BMC Microbiology. 2025;**25**:349. DOI: 10.1186/s12866-025-04076-3

[36] Uzairue LI, Shittu OB, Ojo OE, Obuotor TM, Olanipekun G, Ajose T, et al. Antimicrobial resistance and

virulence genes of invasive *Salmonella enterica* from children with bacteremia in north-Central Nigeria. SAGE Open Medicine. 2023;**11**:20503121231175322. DOI: 10.1177/20503121231175322

[37] Acheampong G, Owusu M, Owusu-Ofori A, Osei I, Sarpong N, Sylverken A, et al. Chromosomal and plasmid-mediated fluoroquinolone resistance in human *Salmonella enterica* infection in Ghana. BMC Infectious Diseases. 2019;**19**:898. DOI: 10.1186/s12879-019-4522-1

[38] Jibril AH, Okeke IN, Dalsgaard A, Olsen JE. Prevalence and whole genome phylogenetic analysis reveal genetic relatedness between antibiotic resistance *Salmonella* in hatchlings and older chickens from farms in Nigeria. Poultry Science. 2023;**102**:102427. DOI: 10.1016/j.psj.2022.102427

[39] Raufu IA, Ahmed OA, Aremu A, Ameh JA, Timme RE, Hendriksen RS, et al. Antimicrobial and genomic characterization of Salmonella Nigeria from pigs and poultry in Ilorin, north-central, Nigeria. Journal of Infection in Developing Countries. 2021a;**15**:1899-1909. DOI: 10.3855/jidc.15025

[40] Shittu OB, Uzairue LI, Ojo OE, Obuotor TM, Folorunso JB, Raheem-Ademola RR, et al. Antimicrobial resistance and virulence genes in *Salmonella enterica* serovars isolated from droppings of layer chicken in two farms in Nigeria. Journal of Applied Microbiology. 2022;**132**:3891-3906. DOI: 10.1111/jam.15477

[41] Somda NS, Savadogo A, Bonkoungou OJI, Wane AA, Zongo C, Traoré Y, et al. First description of the CTX-M9 gene in Salmonella Paratyphi B in Burkina Faso. Médecine et Maladies Infectieuses. 2018;**48**:556-558. DOI: 10.1016/j.medmal.2018.07.007

[42] Kagambèga A, Hiott LM, Boyle DS, McMillan EA, Sharma P, Gupta SK, et al. Serotyping of sub-Saharan Africa Salmonella strains isolated from poultry feces using multiplex PCR and whole genome sequencing. BMC Microbiology. 2021;**21**:29. DOI: 10.1186/s12866-021-02085-6

[43] Akinyemi KO, Fakorede CO, Linde J, Methner U, Wareth G, Tomaso H, et al. Whole genome sequencing of *Salmonella enterica* serovars isolated from humans, animals, and the environment in Lagos, Nigeria. BMC Microbiology. 2023;**23**:164. DOI: 10.1186/s12866-023-02901-1

[44] Raufu IA, Ahmed OA, Aremu A, Ameh JA, Timme RE, Hendriksen RS, et al. Occurrence, antimicrobial resistance and whole genome sequence analysis of Salmonella serovars from pig farms in Ilorin, north-Central Nigeria. International Journal of Food Microbiology. 2021b;**350**:109245. DOI: 10.1016/j.ijfoodmicro.2021.109245

[45] Kagambèga A, Ramadan H, Dione M, Bouda SC, Hiott LM, McMillan EA, et al. Genome analysis of *Salmonella enterica* serovar enteritis strains isolated from poultry and humans in Burkina Faso. Microbiology Resource Announcements. 2024;**13**:e0102423. DOI: 10.1128/mra.01024-23

[46] Useh NM, Ngbede EO, Akange N, Thomas M, Foley A, Keena MC, et al. Draft genome sequences of 37 *Salmonella enterica* strains isolated from poultry sources in Nigeria. Genome Announcements. 2016;**4**:e00315-e00316. DOI: 10.1128/genomeA.00315-16

[47] Zhao J, Lu X, Tie A, Ngegba E, Wang L, Sun L, et al. Molecular diagnostics and next-generation sequencing reveal real etiological characteristics of invasive Salmonella infection in febrile illness in Freetown,

Sierra Leone. Emerging Microbes Infections. 2022;**11**:1416-1424. DOI: 10.1080/22221751.2022.2076612

[48] Vikram A, Jayaprakasha GK, Jesudhasan PR, Pillai SD, Patil BS. Obacunone represses Salmonella pathogenicity islands 1 and 2 in an envZ-dependent fashion. Applied and Environmental Microbiology. 2012;**78**:7012-7022. DOI: 10.1128/AEM.01326-12

[49] Esmael A, Azab E, Gobouri AA, Nasr-Eldin MA, Moustafa MMA, Mohamed SA, et al. Isolation and characterization of two lytic bacteriophages infecting a multi-drug resistant Salmonella typhimurium and their efficacy to combat salmonellosis in ready-to-use foods. Microorganisms. 2021;**9**:423. DOI: 10.3390/microorganisms9020423

[50] Nabil NM, Tawakol MM, Samir A, Hassan HM, Elsayed MM. Evaluation of lyophilized bacteriophage cocktail efficiency against multidrug-resistant Salmonella in broiler chickens. BMC Microbiology. 2024;**24**:338. DOI: 10.1186/s12866-024-03467-2

[51] Torres-Boncompte J, Gómez-Cano IS, Garcia-Llorens J, Soriano JM, Catalá-Gregori P, Sevilla-Navarro S. Characterization and therapeutic potential of newly isolated bacteriophages targeting the most common Salmonella serovars in Europe. Scientific Reports. 2025;**15**:10872. DOI: 10.1038/s41598-025-95398-9

Chapter 2

The Rising Crisis of *Salmonella* Typhimurium in Africa

Derrick A. Daah and Samuel Duodu

Abstract

Non-typhoidal *Salmonella* (NTS) serovars globally cause self-limiting gastroenteritis in healthy humans. While the majority of NTS infections remain localized in the gut, invasive non-typhoidal *Salmonella* (iNTS) serovars have evolved to cause systemic disease. The major contributors of iNTS disease include *Salmonella* Typhimurium, *Salmonella* Enteritidis, and *Salmonella* Dublin. Notably, *S.* Typhimurium sequence type 313 (ST313) and its sublineages have been linked to invasive salmonellosis epidemics, especially in children and the immunocompromised in sub-Saharan Africa (sSA). Unique features of these strains include enhanced survival in host cells and signatures of genome degradation favoring their bloodstream dissemination. Although primarily localized in sSA, ST313 has been detected sporadically in South America and Europe suggesting the potential for global dissemination. The clinical challenges caused by these strains are further exacerbated by their rising antimicrobial resistance, making treatments less effective elevating their threat to public health. This review will examine the burden, biology, evolution, pathogenesis, and antimicrobial resistance of African *S.* Typhimurium. This will shed light on why this pathogen is a pressing public health concern emphasizing the need for continuous research to avert the possibility of global outbreaks of invasive salmonellosis.

Keywords: non-typhoidal *salmonella* (NTS), invasive non-typhoidal *salmonella* (iNTS), *S.* Typhimurium sequence type 313 (ST313), bloodstream infection, multidrug resistance, sub-Saharan Africa

1. Introduction

Salmonella enterica constitutes the largest bacterial species under the genus *Salmonella* with over 2600 serovars identified [1]. The subspecies *enterica* consists of clinically important serovars and is broadly divided into typhoidal and non-typhoidal *Salmonella* (NTS). *Salmonella* Typhi and Paratyphi are the major typhoidal serovars causing typhoid fever in humans. They are host-specific, human restricted and transmitted *via* the fecal oral route. Non-typhoidal *Salmonella* (NTS) serovars have a wide host range and cause self-limiting enterocolitis in the majority of immunocompetent individuals [2]. In these individuals, secondary bacteremia is uncommon and estimated case fatality rates are low [3, 4]. Humans are often infected *via* the fecal-oral route [5–7]. NTS infections can proceed to an invasive infection in infants, children with malaria and malnutrition, and individuals with HIV infections [8]. While the global health trends between 1990 and 2021 show a marked decline in the incidence of typhoid and paratyphoid fever, infections caused by invasive non-typhoidal *Salmonella* (iNTS) have gradually increased during the same period. Although the incidence of typhoid and paratyphoid remains 17 times higher than that of iNTS, the latter now accounts for higher mortality and disability-adjusted life years (DALYs). The rise in iNTS disease burden underscores its significance as a cause of invasive bacterial disease worldwide [9]. Annually, approximately 500,000 cases of iNTS infection are estimated in sSA, with a mean case fatality rate of 14.5%. These figures may be underestimated due to infrequent surveillance and substantial variation in regional and national demographics [10–13]. Typically, iNTS disease is not associated with diarrhea, but presents symptoms of fever, respiratory defects, and hepatosplenomegaly comparable to febrile illnesses such as malaria and typhoid fever [14, 15].

Salmonella enterica serovar Typhimurium (*S.* Typhimurium) is the most common cause of iNTS disease in sub-Saharan Africa (sSA) [16]. While *S.* Typhimurium strains globally responsible for gastroenteritis belong to multilocus sequence types (MLST) ST19 and ST34 [17], those causing bloodstream infections are strongly associated with ST313. These African-associated ST313 strains are broadly classified into distinct lineages (lineages 1 and 2) linked to multidrug resistance [18]. In many countries, ST313 strains are now resistant to commonly used first-line antibiotics such as ampicillin and chloramphenicol [19]. This resistance is believed to be a major driver of the high fatalities associated with iNTS infections [20]. Resistance to second-line antibiotics including ciprofloxacin, ceftriaxone, and azithromycin has also emerged in some African regions [21]. With treatment options narrowing, vaccine development and deployment could serve as promising alternatives. However, no licensed vaccines are currently available to prevent iNTS infections.

This review highlights the emergence and public health implications of invasive *S.* Typhimurium ST313 in sub-Saharan Africa. It synthesizes current knowledge on its pathogenesis and unique genomic characteristics and how it differs from classical NTS strains. Special attention is given to the role of immunosuppressive comorbidities (HIV, malaria) in facilitating the systemic spread of NTS. Additionally highlighted is the increasing antimicrobial resistance of ST313 and the slow progress in iNTS vaccine development. By bringing these elements together, the review underscores the urgency of surveillance, therapeutic innovation, and prevention strategies tailored toward the African population.

2. Epidemiology and burden of iNTS

In 2021, approximately 509,976 new cases of iNTS were reported worldwide. The global age-standardized incidence rate (ASIR), which adjusts for differences in population age structure to allow for fair comparisons, was 7.21 per 100,000 people. However, sSA far exceeded this global average, reflecting a disproportionate concentration of the disease burden. Western and Central sSA continued to report consistently high iNTS incidence and DALY rates. The number of new cases of iNTS in the Western regions surged to 305,959 in 2021 alone with an estimated ASIR of 47.54 per 100,000 population, which is more than six times the global average [22].

At the national level, several African countries emerged as key hotspots. Nigeria reported the highest absolute numbers in 2021, with approximately 164,230 incident cases, 21,614 deaths, and over 1.75 million DALYs attributed to iNTS. In contrast, Mali, while having a smaller total number of cases, recorded the highest rates relative to its population. Mali's incidence rate was estimated at 107.44 per 100,000, its death rate at 16.6 per 100,000, and carried a similarly high DALY burden. These national figures highlight the geographic variability in iNTS burden within Africa and point to the need for country-specific responses.

The disease burden is highest among infants under 1 year old. This group exhibits the most elevated rates of infection, death, and DALY loss [22]. Children in this age group are particularly vulnerable due to underdeveloped immune systems and increased exposure to risk factors such as malnutrition and malaria that are widespread in many African regions.

3. Pathogenesis of NTS

3.1 Microbiota-mediated defense against NTS colonization

To cause disease, NTS must overcome the complex environment of the gastrointestinal tract, which is influenced by the microbiome, immune system, and dietary factors. Colonization resistance (CR), a microbiota-mediated defense process, is mediated by a range of strategies that restrict pathogen survival and proliferation within the gastrointestinal tract [23]. These include the production of antimicrobial agents such as bacteriocins and colicins, which directly inhibit pathogen growth. Physical competition for binding sites on the epithelial and mucus surfaces further prevents pathogen colonization. Additionally, the gut microbiota lowers oxygen availability in the intestine, creating conditions that suppress facultative anaerobic pathogens like NTS. Commensals also reduce pathogen fitness by competing for essential nutrients. *Escherichia coli* has been shown to restrict NTS infection by limiting access to electron acceptors like fumarate and carbon sources such as galactitol necessary for its proliferation [24, 25]. Recent findings have identified nociceptor sensory neurons, known for their role in detecting noxious stimuli, as important contributors to CR against NTS [26].

3.2 NTS proliferation in the gastrointestinal tract

NTS can proliferate in the large intestine when environmental conditions are favorable, and CR is not a barrier. This growth is supported by secretion systems encoded within *Salmonella* pathogenicity islands (SPIs). SPIs are commonly introduced into the genome *via* horizontal gene transfer and are subsequently integrated and stably maintained within the bacterial chromosome [27–29]. NTS utilizes the type VI secretion system (T6SS) to outcompete bacterial competitors by their elimination through dependent and independent mechanisms [30]. In the contact dependent pathway, NTS uses the T6SS to deliver toxic effector proteins directly into target cells [31]. On the other hand, in the contact independent mechanism, effectors are secreted into the extracellular medium. Through this mechanism, NTS competes for essential nutrients such as iron by producing siderophores including enterobactin and salmochelin [32]. Once these defenses are overcome, NTS multiplies rapidly, reaching high bacterial densities within the gut.

3.3 Invasion of epithelial cells by NTS

Attachment of NTS to epithelial cells is mediated by fimbrial and non-fimbrial adhesins [33]. Once attached, *Salmonella* employs the Trigger and Zipper mechanisms for invasion of cells. The "Trigger" mechanism, driven by T3SS-1 effectors such as SopB, SopE, and SopE2, induces dramatic actin cytoskeletal rearrangements forming membrane ruffles that lead to NTS internalization into epithelial cells [34, 35]. Additionally, the effectors SipA and SipC promote invasion by directly nucleating and bundling actin filaments [36–38]. The "Zipper" mechanism depends on the outer membrane proteins Rck and PagN. These proteins activate the phosphatidylinositol 3-kinase (PI3K) signaling cascade by binding to host receptors like EGFR. This causes cytoskeletal rearrangements that facilitate bacterial uptake [39]. However, NTS strains lacking Rck, PagN, and T3SS-1 still efficiently invade fibroblasts, epithelial, and endothelial cells, implying the presence of yet undiscovered invasion mechanisms [40].

3.4 NTS intracellular persistence and resistance to inflammatory responses

Upon infection, host cells respond by activating inflammasomes and inducing pyroptosis. This defense mechanism commences with the NAIP/NLRC4 inflammasome, which recognizes bacterial protein ligands such as flagellin and the T3SS needle protein PrgI, leading to the release of IL-18 and subsequent IFNγ production [41, 42]. NTS overcomes this response by residing within *Salmonella*-containing vacuoles (SCVs) intracellularly. Inhibition of autophagy, mediated by T3SS-2 effectors, additionally facilitates the intracellular survival of NTS. These effector proteins deubiquitinate SCVs, thereby reducing autophagy markers p62 and LC3 [43]. The formation of autophagosomes is further prevented by SseF and SseG, which disrupt Rab1A signaling [44] by SpvC through its phosphothreonine lyase activity [45] and by SpvB (from the pSLT plasmid), which depolymerizes the actin [46].

NTS further impairs the functions of cells of the immune system which include macrophages and dendritic cells (DC). Macrophages are crucial for phagocytosing NTS post-epithelial breach. They can exist in M1 (pathogen-killing) and M2 (tissue repair) forms [47]. The T3SS-2 effector SteE skews macrophages toward an M2 phenotype, enhancing NTS survival [48]. Macrophage-produced lactate additionally induces T3SS-2 and SteE translocation, promoting this shift [49]. DC function is also affected by NTS. The T3SS-2 effector SteD degrades mature MHC-II, impairing antigen presentation to CD4+ T cells. This disrupts dendritic cell-T cell interactions leading to a diminished T-cell response [50, 51].

4. Transition from NTS to iNTS

The ability of NTS to breach the intestinal epithelium and establish systemic infection is closely linked to immunosuppression as iNTS is rarely observed in otherwise healthy individuals. Consequently, current understanding of iNTS pathogenesis is largely drawn from studies involving immunocompromised populations. In this section, we explore how NTS co-infections with malaria and HIV create permissive environments for the transition of NTS to iNTS offering insights into the mechanisms underlying iNTS pathogenesis.

4.1 iNTS and malaria

Malaria and invasive non-typhoidal *Salmonella* (iNTS) infections are prevalent in sSA where their geographical distributions frequently coincide [52]. This risk is most prevalent in children with severe malarial anemia (SMA) [53]. In rural areas with high malaria transmission, NTS is frequently the main bacteria isolated from the bloodstream of children with *Plasmodium* parasitemia [54, 55]. Moreover, public health measures that reduce malaria incidence have often led to a parallel decrease in NTS bacteremia cases, an effect not consistently seen with other bacterial infections [56, 57].

4.1.1 Malaria as a cause of NTS systemic dissemination

Hemolysis is a defining characteristic of malaria infections [57]. This extensive destruction of red blood cells during malaria releases large amounts of hemoglobin and free heme, which increases the availability of iron, essential for *Salmonella* growth and multiplication. Macrophages ingest these damaged red cells and become overloaded with iron. This iron-rich intracellular environment within macrophages can support the survival and replication of ingested NTS [58, 59]. SMA is associated with reduced hepcidin levels, a hormone that regulates iron availability. Lower hepcidin levels allow more iron to be available within the SCV, promoting bacterial growth. This mechanism highlights how malaria indirectly supports NTS proliferation by altering iron homeostasis [60].

Gut barrier dysfunction is a mechanism facilitating the susceptibility of malaria-infected individuals to NTS infections. Sequestration of parasitized red blood cells in the gut's microvasculature triggers inflammation, hypoxia, and disruption of tight junctions between intestinal epithelial cells. This compromises the intestinal barrier integrity causing the translocation of enteric bacteria, including NTS, from the gut lumen into the bloodstream [61, 62]. Additionally, malaria-associated deficiency of L-arginine has been linked to increased intestinal mast cell activity, histamine release, and enhanced intestinal permeability [63]. Malaria compromises the host's ability to resist enteric pathogens by reducing gastric acidity. Studies have shown that *Plasmodium yoelii* infection in mice elevates gastric pH, creating a less acidic environment that facilitates the survival and colonization of *S.* Typhimurium in the upper gastrointestinal tract [64].

Overall epidemiological and biological evidence strongly supports a relationship where malaria increases susceptibility to iNTS disease.

4.2 iNTS and HIV

Prior to the widespread availability of antiretroviral therapy (ART) in sSA, iNTS was recognized as one of the most common causes of bloodstream infections among HIV-infected adults and children [65, 66]. Incidence rates were reported to be 20- to 100-fold higher in HIV-infected individuals compared to their HIV-uninfected counterparts in the same communities [67]. This disparity underscored HIV as a primary risk factor for invasive disease. A critical feature of iNTS in the HIV-infected population is the high rate of recurrent bacteremia, often with the same NTS strain, suggesting incomplete bacterial clearance or persistence [68].

4.2.1 HIV as a cause of systemic NTS infections

The hallmark of HIV infection is the progressive depletion and functional impairment of CD4+ T-lymphocytes [69]. These cells, particularly T-helper 1 (Th1) and T-helper 17 (Th17) subsets, are vital for effective immunity against intracellular pathogens like *Salmonella*. Th1 cells produce IFN-γ, a cytokine essential for activating macrophages to kill intracellular *Salmonella*. Th17 cells contribute to maintaining mucosal barrier integrity and recruiting neutrophils to sites of infection [70]. HIV preferentially infects and depletes Th17 cells, especially within the gut-associated lymphoid tissue (GALT), the primary site of *Salmonella* invasion [71]. Their loss contributes to increased intestinal permeability, facilitating the translocation of *Salmonella* and other microbial products from the intestinal lumen into the systemic circulation, thereby promoting bacteremia [72].

HIV infection compromises multiple macrophage functions *via* the depletion of Th1 cells. Macrophages from people living with HIV/AIDS (PLWH) may exhibit reduced phagocytic capacity, impaired oxidative burst, and deficient production of pro-inflammatory cytokines such as TNF-α in response to *Salmonella* infection [2]. Antibodies, particularly secretory IgA (sIgA) at mucosal surfaces and serum IgG, play a significant role in controlling *Salmonella*. HIV infection leads to B-cell dysregulation, resulting in impaired production of antibodies against various pathogens [73]. Studies have demonstrated that HIV-infected individuals often have lower levels of *Salmonella*-specific antibodies and reduced opsonophagocytic activity, which are critical for preventing bacteremia [74]. This defect in antibody-mediated immunity is considered a major contributor to the high incidence of iNTS.

Collectively, these immunological defects create a permissive environment for *Salmonella* to breach mucosal defenses, disseminate systemically, survive within host cells, and evade clearance, leading to the severe and often recurrent iNTS disease observed in PLWH.

5. Pathoadaptive features underpinning ST313-mediated iNTS in Africa

The burden and distribution of iNTS in Africa raises important questions about pathogen-specific factors that may amplify disease severity. While host factors are crucial in determining susceptibility to iNTS infections, they do not fully explain why only certain NTS strains cause systemic infections. Recent studies have revealed that the dominant *S.* Typhimurium ST313 strains circulating in sSA differ markedly from globally prevalent non-invasive strains like ST19. The following section explores these differences and how they may contribute to the unique disease profile observed in the region. Understanding how these strains differ from classical *S.* Typhimurium lineages is crucial to grasping the full landscape of iNTS pathogenesis.

5.1 Unique genetic composition of ST313

The enhanced systemic survival of ST313 appears tightly linked to its distinct genetic architecture. Comparative genomics has revealed that ST313 harbors numerous pseudogenes, deletions, and prophage elements absent in non-invasive strains. A defining feature of ST313 lineage 2 is the acquisition of two unique prophages—BTP1 and BTP5—which are absent from ST19 and ST313 isolates from outside Africa [75, 76]. BTP1 encodes the *st313-td* gene, which enhances intracellular replication in macrophages [77]. Another element, the *gtrAC* operon, encodes glycosyltransferases that modify the structure and length of the O-antigen (OAg), a critical determinant of resistance to antibody-mediated killing. ST313 OAg chains are typically longer, conferring serum resistance, a hallmark of systemic pathogenesis [75, 78, 79]. Furthermore, ST313 strains display a unique single nucleotide polymorphism (SNP) in the promoter of the *pgtE* gene, leading to its upregulation. *pgtE* encodes an outer membrane protease that disrupts the host complement system by degrading complement proteins, enhancing survival in serum [80]. Intriguingly, this same mutation is also present in *S.* Gallinarum and upregulation of pgtE has been noted during *S.* Typhi infection of human macrophages suggesting convergent evolution toward an invasive phenotype [81]. ST313 has undergone additional functional losses in genes associated with metabolic flexibility and gastrointestinal persistence. Inactivating mutations have been reported in genes such as *allB, allP, ttdA, melR, ratB,* and *macAB*, many of which are intact in ST19 [76, 82, 83]. These mutations likely reduce the bacterium's ability to persist in the gut, in favor of systemic dissemination. Moreover, genes essential for iron acquisition and siderophore secretion are repressed in ST313 than in ST19 [82]. This could reflect a metabolic adaptation to iron-rich environments, such as macrophages co-infected with malaria parasites, where iron availability is increased [84].

5.2 Accumulation of pseudogenes

The gradual pseudogenization of specific genes provides further evidence of host adaptation. ST313 strains have accumulated numerous pseudogenes. In the genome of the ST313 D23580 strain, 77 pseudogenes have been observed out of which 23 are strain specific [18, 82, 85]. This mirrors patterns observed in host-adapted serovars such as *S.* Gallinarum, *S.* Typhi, and *S.* Paratyphi, which carry numerous pseudogenes as they shed functions unnecessary for systemic survival [86–89]. One recently characterized pseudogene in ST313 is *sseI*, which encodes an effector of the SPI-2 type III secretion system (T3SS). In functional form, *sseI* promotes the inhibition of DC chemotaxis. Inactivation of *sseI* results in hyper-dissemination of DCs to lymph nodes in murine models, thereby facilitating systemic spread [90]. Furthermore, the downregulation of the SPI-1 effector sopE2 is commonly observed in ST313 isolates and correlates with reduced epithelial invasion [91]. Notably, *sopE2* is also pseudogenized in *S.* Typhi [81] suggesting functional convergence with other invasive serovars. Similarly, deletions in *pipD,* a gene implicated in intestinal fluid accumulation, contribute to reduced intestinal inflammation in ST313 lineage 2 [83].

6. Transmission and reservoir dynamics of ST313

Understanding the reservoir and transmission routes of iNTS has remained a challenge since its emergence as a major cause of blood stream infections in sSA [19]. This in contrast to NTS infections that are predominantly transmitted *via* zoonotic and foodborne pathways [92]. Early investigations in Kenya and The Gambia failed to identify a consistent animal or environmental source for iNTS. The limited sample sizes and narrow geographic focus may have contributed to this uncertainty [93, 94]. Experimentally, ST313 has been shown to colonize the chicken gut and invade systemic sites, though less efficiently than the gastroenteritis causing NTS serovars [95]. Despite the isolation of other invasive *Salmonella* serovars from livestock, slaughterhouses, and retail meat, ST313 has not been detected in these samples [96]. So far, ST313 is isolated exclusively from human sources. Genomic analysis showed low diversity across isolates, consistent with host adaptation and restriction supporting a pattern of continuous human-to-human spread. The absence of environmental or animal detections, coupled with evidence of asymptomatic fecal shedding among humans, strengthens the argument for anthroponotic transmission as recently reported [97].

A clearer definition of the transmission dynamics is essential for understanding ST313 evolution and guiding public health action. If human-to-human transmission proves dominant, interventions must prioritize vaccine development, sanitation infrastructure, and identification of chronic carriers. Conversely, confirmation of an animal reservoir would necessitate strategies focused on food safety and animal vaccination. Clarifying these routes is central to designing targeted measures against iNTS infections in Africa.

7. The escalating antimicrobial resistance crisis of ST313 in Africa

A defining hallmark of this pathogen is its continual accumulation of antimicrobial resistance (AMR), progressively rendering treatment regimens ineffective. Geographically distinct sublineages, such as sublineage 2.2 in Malawi [98] and extensively drug resistant (XDR) ST313 strains in the DRC [99], reflect local adaptation under antibiotic pressure. Surveillance studies from Nigeria [100], Zambia [101], The Gambia [102], Mozambique [103], and Sierra Leone [104] confirm the widespread presence and expanding resistance of ST313. This section explores the resistance profile of ST313, illustrating the genetic mechanisms underpinning the evolution and the clinical challenges it poses across Africa.

7.1 Resistance to first-line antimicrobial classes

ST313 is currently resistant to all three first-line antimicrobial classes traditionally used for iNTS infections: beta-lactams (ampicillin), phenicols (chloramphenicol), and folate pathway inhibitors (trimethoprim-sulfamethoxazole) [14, 105]. Beta-lactam resistance in ST313 is largely conferred by the plasmid-encoded *bla*TEM-1B gene, while *catA1* mediates chloramphenicol resistance. The *catA* gene, located on a pSTm-ST313-II.1 plasmid, encodes chloramphenicol acetyltransferase, which enzymatically inactivates the antibiotic. Resistance to trimethoprim-sulfamethoxazole is driven by the combined action of *dfrA* genes that encode dihydrofolate reductase and sulfonamide resistance genes (*sul1*, *sul2*). These are commonly embedded within class 1 integrons housed on IncHI1 plasmids such as pBT1 [99, 106, 107].

7.2 Resistance to second-line antimicrobial agents

In response to first-line treatment failure, clinicians shifted to fluoroquinolones (e.g., ciprofloxacin) and third-generation cephalosporins (e.g., ceftriaxone). However, ST313 isolates have evolved resistance to these agents [16, 108]. Fluoroquinolone resistance arises from point mutations in the quinolone resistance-determining regions (QRDRs) of *gyrA*, *gyrB*, *parC*, and *parE*. Notably, nonsynonymous substitutions such as *gyrA* Ser83 → Phe and Asp87 → Asn are commonly observed in resistant isolates from Africa [99, 100]. Ceftriaxone resistance has arisen due to the acquisition and dissemination of extended-spectrum beta-lactamases (ESBLs), particularly *bla*CTX-M-15, often carried on IncN and IncI1 plasmids [99, 101, 107]. These mobile elements frequently co-localize with other resistance determinants, enabling co-selection and persistence of ESBL genes even in the absence of direct cephalosporin exposure.

7.3 Expansion of resistance into additional antimicrobial classes

Considering the declining efficacy of second-line agents, azithromycin has been employed as an alternative. However, resistance to macrolides is now emerging. This development is particularly evident in XDR ST313 lineages identified in the Democratic Republic of Congo (DRC). Azithromycin is often a last-resort oral antibiotic in regions with limited intravenous options. The emergence of azithromycin resistance in ST313 poses a threat to the continued use of azithromycin, which is one of the few remaining oral options for empirical treatment in children and outpatients. ST313 has also acquired resistance to aminoglycosides. Genes such as *aadA1* and *aadA2* encode aminoglycoside-modifying enzymes that inactivate gentamicin, streptomycin, and amikacin [99, 106]. The accumulation of these resistance determinants has led to near-total resistance to all commonly available antibiotics in some regions.

7.4 Public health implications and strategic interventions

Combating ST313's resistance crisis demands integrated approaches. Enhanced genomic surveillance is critical for monitoring resistance patterns and informing antimicrobial policy. Stewardship programs are urgently needed to curb antibiotic misuse in human and veterinary medicine. Vaccine development against ST313 and other iNTS serovars is progressing at various stages of development [109–111]. Ultimately, addressing the AMR crisis caused by ST313 will require a One Health approach that unifies efforts across human, animal, and environmental health domains.

8. Vaccine progress toward elimination of ST313

The MDR phenotype of ST313 has rendered antibiotic therapy ineffective, creating an urgent need for prevention strategies. Currently, no licensed vaccines specifically targeting iNTS serovars are currently available. This is in sharp contrast to the availability of vaccines targeting typhoidal *Salmonella* serovars (Vi-polysaccharide conjugate vaccines) [112]. It is predicted that, without vaccination, iNTS mortality will climb significantly especially among the immunocompromised. Studies suggests that effective vaccine deployment could avert over 70% of these deaths and curb iNTS transmission [109]. The global effort to develop a vaccine against iNTS has yielded vaccine candidates, with several demonstrating compelling safety and immunogenicity in human trials. The following section will explore the merits, progress, and challenges of the leading vaccine candidates that represent the forefront of the global effort to control iNTS infections.

8.1 Live-attenuated vaccines

Live-attenuated vaccines, which utilize a weakened version of the pathogen to mimic natural infection, represent a foundational approach in *Salmonella* vaccinology. Its primary advantage is the ability to induce a broad spectrum of immune responses [113]. Early human studies explored strains with deletions in key virulence-regulating gene systems like phoP/phoQ [114] or those with defined auxotrophic mutations in essential metabolic pathways, such as *aroC*, and virulence systems, like *ssaV* [115].

Newer approaches, including radiation mutation enhancement technology [116] and the creation of auxotrophic live vaccines [117], have shown significant efficacy in preclinical models. Despite these advances, human clinical data for live-attenuated iNTS candidates remain limited, and their developmental pathway is currently less advanced.

8.2 Glycoconjugate vaccines

Glycoconjugate vaccines represent one of the most clinically advanced strategies in the iNTS pipeline. A leading example is the trivalent conjugate vaccine platform developed at the University of Maryland, which has progressed through multiple clinical trials. The initial candidate, CVD 1000, paired *S.* Typhimurium and *S.* Enteritidis O-antigens with the Vi polysaccharide from *S.* Typhi. A Phase I trial in adults confirmed its safety and ability to induce sustained IgG titers. An updated formulation, CVD 2000, advanced into Phase II pediatric trials across sSA, demonstrating age-appropriate immune responses in the target infant population [118, 119]. Another significant candidate in this class is the bivalent iNTS OAg-CRM_{197} vaccine, which targets the two most common iNTS serovars. In this approach, the O-antigens of *S.* Typhimurium and *S.* Enteritidis are conjugated to the non-toxic diphtheria toxoid mutant CRM_{197}. CRM_{197} is a carrier protein with a history of safe and effective use in licensed pediatric vaccines [120, 121]. While their complex production and associated costs present potential barriers to access in low-resource settings, the proven ability of glycoconjugate vaccines to elicit protective immunity in infants has set a vital benchmark for all other iNTS vaccine candidates [122, 123].

8.3 Generalized modules for membrane antigens (GMMA)

Vaccines based on Generalized Modules for Membrane Antigens (GMMA) have emerged as an alternative to the glycoconjugate vaccines. GMMA are nanoparticles derived from the outer membrane of genetically engineered bacteria. They are modified to vesicles enriched with key surface antigens, including LPS (containing the O-antigen) and outer membrane proteins (OMPs), in their native conformation. GMMA vaccines possess intrinsic adjuvant properties rendering them potent immunogens, which is a key characteristic of this platform [124, 125]. GMMA vaccines have rapidly progressed into human trials. The Oxford-led SALVO trial confirmed its safety and immunogenicity in healthy adult volunteers [126]. More recently, Phase II studies in Ghana as part of the PEDVAC-iNTS consortium have shown the iNTS-GMMA vaccine demonstrates good tolerability and elicits prolonged antigen-specific IgG responses in children and infants [127, 128]. By combining potent immunogenicity with a favorable manufacturing profile, the GMMA platform is argued to be strongly positioned to deliver an effective and accessible vaccine.

8.4 Multiple antigen presentation system (MAPS)

The Multiple Antigen Presentation System (MAPS) platform offers an innovative approach to creating multivalent vaccines. This technology utilizes a dextran backbone to which multiple antigens can be attached *via* a high-affinity, non-covalent biotin–rhizavidin linkage. This design allows for the presentation of a diverse array of antigens in a single formulation, stimulating broad immunity [129]. A quadrivalent MAPS vaccine targeting *S.* Typhimurium, *S.* Enteritidis, *S.* Typhi, and *S.* Paratyphi A has been shown to confer broad protective immunity in preclinical models after just two doses [130]. Given the frequent co-circulation of typhoidal and iNTS serovars, multivalent vaccines are strategic in the elimination of the major causes of febrile illnesses in sSA. The global effort to develop a vaccine against iNTS has yielded a rich and advanced pipeline of candidates, with several demonstrating compelling safety and immunogenicity in human trials. The journey from a promising vaccine candidate to a widely implemented public health tool requires a clear strategic vision that addresses both regulatory and economic challenges in populations at risk.

9. Conclusion

The persistence of ST313 in sSA underscores the need for effective control, prevention, and policy formulation. While the burden of ST313 has been established, uncertainties remain regarding its ecological dynamics, host-pathogen interactions, and its evolution. Although current evidence suggests human-to-human transmission of ST313, the role of environmental or zoonotic reservoirs has not been adequately addressed. Many existing studies are geographically limited and lack sufficient sampling depth to definitively rule out the contribution of livestock, contaminated water sources, or foodborne pathways. Increased surveillance using One Health approach is therefore essential to clarify ST313's transmission routes and inform multisectoral intervention strategies. Equally underexplored is the immunological response to ST313 in high-risk populations. Infants, individuals living with HIV, and patients co-infected with malaria represent the most affected groups. Studies targeting these populations are required to ensure that vaccine candidates are both immunogenic and protective. The pathogen's ongoing evolution also demands closer attention. ST313 continues to acquire multidrug resistance while undergoing genomic adaptations associated with enhanced intracellular survival and immune evasion. However, genomic surveillance of iNTS serovars remains limited across sSA. This poses a potential danger of novel resistant or hypervirulent strains going undetected. Integrating sequencing into national and regional surveillance efforts will help guide treatment, inform vaccine development, and support public health responses. Although ST313 has been described as an African confined iNTS serovar, recent isolations in the United Kingdom, Brazil, and other non-endemic regions indicate that it is no longer geographically restricted. Timely interventions are therefore required in stemming the international spread of ST313 to mitigate the possibility of global outbreaks of iNTS infections.

Author contributions

Both authors contributed to this summary on the rising crisis of *Salmonella* Typhimurium in Africa and have read and agreed to the published version of the manuscript.

Funding

This research was supported by WACCBIP, University of Ghana, which receives funding from World Bank African Centre of Excellence (WACCBIP + NCDs, Awandare).

Conflict of interest

The authors declare no conflict of interest.

Author details

Derrick A. Daah[1,2] and Samuel Duodu[1,2]*

1 Department of Biochemistry, Cell and Molecular Biology, University of Ghana, Accra, Ghana

2 West African Centre for Cell Biology of Infectious Pathogens, University of Ghana, Accra, Ghana

*Address all correspondence to: saduodu@ug.edu.gh

References

[1] Issenhuth-Jeanjean S, Roggentin P, Mikoleit M, Guibourdenche M, De Pinna E, Nair S, et al. Supplement 2008-2010 (no. 48) to the White–Kauffmann–Le minor scheme. Research in Microbiology. 2014;**165**(7):526-530

[2] Hohmann EL. Nontyphoidal salmonellosis. Clinical Infectious Diseases. 2001;**32**:263-269

[3] Voetsch AC, Gilder TJ, Angulo FJ, Farley MM, Shallow S, Marcus R, et al. FoodNet estimate of the burden of illness caused by nontyphoidal Salmonella infections in the United States. Clinical Infectious Diseases. 2004;**38**(Suppl. 3): 127-134

[4] Adak GK, Long SM, O'Brien SJ. Trends in indigenous foodborne disease and deaths. Gut. 2002;**51**:832-841

[5] Angulo FJ. A community waterborne outbreak of salmonellosis and the effectiveness of a boil water order. American Journal of Public Health. 1997;**87**:580-584

[6] Mishu B. Outbreaks of *Salmonella enteritidis* infections in the United States, 1985-1991. Journal of Infectious Diseases. 1994;**169**:547-552

[7] Majowicz SE. The global burden of nontyphoidal Salmonella gastroenteritis. Clinical Infectious Diseases. 2010;**50**:882-889

[8] Okoro CK, Kingsley RA, Connor TR, Harris SR, Parry CM, Al-Mashhadani MN, et al. Intracontinental spread of human invasive *Salmonella typhimurium* pathovariants in sub-Saharan Africa. Nature Genetics. 2012;**44**(11):1215-1221

[9] Shi K, You T. Global trends in typhoid and paratyphoid, and invasive non-typhoidal salmonella, and the burden of antimicrobial resistance: A trend analysis study from 1990 to 2021. Frontiers in Medicine (Lausanne). 2025;**12**:1588507

[10] Ao TT, Daugla DM, Toralta J, Ngadoua C, Fermon F, Page AL, et al. Global burden of invasive nontyphoidal *Salmonella* disease. Emerging Infectious Diseases. 2015;**21**(6):941-949

[11] Stanaway JD, Parisi A, Sarkar K, Blacker BF, Reiner RC, Hay SI, et al. The global burden of non-typhoidal *Salmonella* invasive disease: A systematic analysis for the global burden of disease study 2017. The Lancet Infectious Diseases. 2019;**19**(12):1312-1324

[12] Reddy EA, Shaw AV, Crump JA. Community-acquired bloodstream infections in Africa: A systematic review and meta-analysis. The Lancet Infectious Diseases. 2010;**10**(6):417-432

[13] Hendriksen RS, Vieira AR, Karlsmose S, Lo Fo Wong DMA, Jensen AB, Wegener HC, et al. Global monitoring of *Salmonella* serovar distribution from the world health organization global foodborne infections network country data bank: Results of quality assured laboratories from 2001 to 2007. Foodborne Pathogens and Disease. 2011;**8**(8):887-900

[14] Crump JA, Heyderman RS. A perspective on invasive *Salmonella* disease in Africa. Clinical Infectious Diseases. 2015;**61**:S235-S240

[15] Uche IV, MacLennan CA, Saul A. A systematic review of the incidence, risk factors and case fatality rates of invasive nontyphoidal *Salmonella* (iNTS) disease in Africa (1966 to 2014). PLoS Neglected Tropical Diseases. 2017;**11**(1):1-28

[16] Kariuki S, Gordon MA, Feasey N, Parry CM. Antimicrobial resistance and management of invasive *Salmonella* disease. Vaccine. 2015;**33**(S3):21-29

[17] Alikhan NF, Zhou Z, Sergeant MJ, Achtman M. A genomic overview of the population structure of *Salmonella*. PLoS Genetics. 2018;**14**(4):e1007261

[18] Kingsley RA, Msefula CL, Thomson NR, Kariuki S, Holt KE, Gordon MA, et al. Epidemic multiple drug resistant *Salmonella typhimurium* causing invasive disease in sub-Saharan Africa have a distinct genotype. Genome Research. 2009;**19**(12):2279-2287

[19] Kariuki S, Revathi G, Kariuki N, Kiiru J, Mwituria J, Muyodi J, et al. Invasive multidrug-resistant non-typhoidal *Salmonella* infections in Africa: Zoonotic or anthroponotic transmission? Journal of Medical Microbiology. 2006;**55**(5):585-591

[20] Marchello CS, Birkhold M, Crump JA, Martin LB, Ansah MO, Breghi G, et al. Complications and mortality of non-typhoidal *Salmonella* invasive disease: A global systematic review and meta-analysis. The Lancet Infectious Diseases. 2022;**22**(5):692-705

[21] Tack B, Vanaenrode J, Verbakel JY, Toelen J, Jacobs J. Invasive non-typhoidal *Salmonella* infections in sub-Saharan Africa: A systematic review on antimicrobial resistance and treatment. BMC Medicine. 2020;**18**(1):212

[22] He Y, Jia Q, Cai K, Xu S, Li H, Xie Q, et al. The global, regional, and national burden of invasive non-typhoidal *Salmonella* (iNTS): An analysis from the global burden of disease study 1990-2021. PLoS Neglected Tropical Diseases. 2025;**19**(4):e0012960

[23] Stecher B. Establishing causality in *Salmonella*-microbiota-host interaction: The use of gnotobiotic mouse models and synthetic microbial communities. International Journal of Medical Microbiology [Internet]. 2021;**311**(3):151484. Available from: https://www.sciencedirect.com/science/article/pii/S1438422121000138 [Accessed: June 18, 2025]

[24] Nguyen BD, Cuenca VM, Hartl J, Gül E, Bauer R, Meile S, et al. Import of aspartate and malate by DcuABC drives H2/fumarate respiration to promote initial *Salmonella* gut-lumen colonization in mice. Cell Host & Microbe. 2020;**27**(6):922-936.e6

[25] Eberl C, Weiss AS, Jochum LM, Durai Raj AC, Ring D, Hussain S, et al. *E. coli* enhance colonization resistance against *Salmonella typhimurium* by competing for galactitol, a context-dependent limiting carbon source. Cell Host & Microbe. 2021;**29**(11):1680-1692.e7

[26] Lai NY, Musser MA, Pinho-Ribeiro FA, Baral P, Jacobson A, Ma P, et al. Gut-innervating nociceptor neurons regulate Peyer's patch microfold cells and SFB levels to mediate *Salmonella* host defense. Cell. 2020;**180**(1):33-49.e22

[27] Hensel M. Evolution of pathogenicity islands of *Salmonella enterica*. International Journal of Medical Microbiology. 2004;**294**(2-3):95-102

[28] Schmidt H, Hensel M. Pathogenicity islands in bacterial pathogenesis. Clinical Microbiology Reviews. 2004;**17**(1):14-56

[29] Roer L, Hendriksen RS, Leekitcharoenphon P, Lukjancenko O, Kaas RS, Hasman H, et al. Is the evolution of *Salmonella enterica* subsp. *Enterica* linked to restriction-modification systems? mSystems. 2016;**1**(3):e00009-e00016

[30] Blondel CJ, Amaya FA, Reyes-Méndez F, Soriano-Mora V,

Vargas C, Parra A, et al. Deciphering the *Salmonella* T6SS toolkit: Two decades of research decoding a versatile bacterial weapon. Journal of Bacteriology. 2025;**207**(7):e00188-25

[31] Coulthurst S. The type VI secretion system: A versatile bacterial weapon. Microbiology (United Kingdom). 2019;**165**(5):503-515

[32] Mohsen Y, Tarchichi N, Barakat R, Kawtharani I, Ghandour R, Ezzeddine Z, et al. The different types of metallophores produced by *Salmonella enterica*: A review. Microbiology Research. 2023;**14**(3):1457-1469

[33] Bao H, Wang S, Zhao JH, Liu SL. *Salmonella* secretion systems: Differential roles in pathogen-host interactions. Microbiological Research [Internet]. 2020;**241**:126591. Available from: https://www.sciencedirect.com/science/article/pii/S0944501320304596 [Accessed: June 18, 2025]

[34] Fredlund J, Santos JC, Stévenin V, Weiner A, Latour-Lambert P, Rechav K, et al. The entry of *Salmonella* in a distinct tight compartment revealed at high temporal and ultrastructural resolution. Cellular Microbiology. 2018;**20**(4). DOI: 10.1111/cmi.12816

[35] Koczerka M, Lantier I, Morillon M, Deperne J, Clamagirand CD, Virlogeux-Payant I, et al. From intestine to beyond: *Salmonella* entry factors display distinct transcription pattern upon infection in murine models. Open Biology. 2024;**14**(1):230312

[36] McGhie EJ, Hayward RD, Koronakis V. Cooperation between actin-binding proteins of invasive *Salmonella*: SipA potentiates SipC nucleation and bundling of actin. EMBO Journal [Internet]. 2001;**20**(9):2131-2139. DOI: 10.1093/emboj/20.9.2131?download=true

[37] Humphreys D, Davidson A, Hume PJ, Koronakis V. *Salmonella* virulence effector SopE and host GEF ARNO cooperate to recruit and activate WAVE to trigger bacterial invasion. Cell Host & Microbe. 2012;**11**(2):129-139

[38] Fattinger SA, Sellin ME, Hardt WD. *Salmonella* effector driven invasion of the gut epithelium: Breaking in and setting the house on fire. Current Opinion in Microbiology. 2021;**64**:9-18

[39] Barilleau E, Védrine M, Koczerka M, Burlaud-Gaillard J, Kempf F, Grépinet O, et al. Investigation of the invasion mechanism mediated by the outer membrane protein PagN of *Salmonella typhimurium*. BMC Microbiology. 2021;**21**(1):1-18

[40] Rosselin M, Abed N, Virlogeux-Payant I, Bottreau E, Sizaret PY, Velge P, et al. Heterogeneity of type III secretion system (T3SS)-1-independent entry mechanisms used by *Salmonella enteritidis* to invade different cell types. Microbiology (N Y). 2011;**157**(3):839-847

[41] Gram AM, Wright JA, Pickering RJ, Lam NL, Booty LM, Webster SJ, et al. *Salmonella flagellin* activates NAIP/NLRC4 and canonical NLRP3 inflammasomes in human macrophages. The Journal of Immunology [Internet]. 2021;**206**(3):631-640. DOI: 10.4049/jimmunol.2000382

[42] Pandeya A, Zhang Y, Cui J, Yang L, Li J, Zhang G, et al. Inflammasome activation and pyroptosis mediate coagulopathy and inflammation in *Salmonella* systemic infection. Microbiological Research. 2023;**275**:127460

[43] Mesquita FS, Thomas M, Sachse M, Santos AJM, Figueira R, Holden DW. The *Salmonella* deubiquitinase SseI inhibits selective autophagy of

cytosolic aggregates. PLoS Pathogens. 2012;**8**(6):e1002743

[44] Feng ZZ, Jiang AJ, Mao AW, Feng Y, Wang W, Li J, et al. The *Salmonella* effectors SseF and SseG inhibit Rab1A-mediated autophagy to facilitate intracellular bacterial survival and replication. Journal of Biological Chemistry. 2018;**293**(25):9662-9673

[45] Zhou L, Li Y, Gao S, Yuan H, Zuo L, Wu C, et al. *Salmonella* spvC gene inhibits autophagy of host cells and suppresses NLRP3 as well as NLRC4. Frontiers in Immunology. 2021;**12**:639019

[46] Chu Y, Gao S, Wang T, Yan J, Xu G, Li Y, et al. A novel contribution of spvB to pathogenesis of *Salmonella typhimurium* by inhibiting autophagy in host cells. Oncotarget. 2016;**7**(7):8295

[47] Brodsky IE. JAK-ing into M1/M2 polarization SteErs *Salmonella*-containing macrophages away from immune attack to promote bacterial persistence. Cell Host & Microbe. 2020;**27**(1):3-5

[48] Panagi I, Jennings E, Zeng J, Günster RA, Stones CD, Mak H, et al. *Salmonella* effector SteE converts the mammalian serine/threonine kinase GSK3 into a tyrosine kinase to direct macrophage polarization. Cell Host & Microbe. 2020;**27**(1):41-53.e6

[49] Wang X, Yang B, Ma S, Yan X, Ma S, Sun H, et al. Lactate promotes *Salmonella* intracellular replication and systemic infection via driving macrophage M2 polarization. Microbiology Spectrum. 2023;**11**(6):e02253-23

[50] Alix E, Godlee C, Cerny O, Blundell S, Tocci R, Matthews S, et al. The tumour suppressor TMEM127 is a Nedd4-family E3 ligase adaptor required by *Salmonella* SteD to Ubiquitinate and degrade MHC class II molecules. Cell Host & Microbe. 2020;**28**(1):54-68.e7

[51] Cerny O, Godlee C, Tocci R, Cross NE, Shi H, Williamson JC, et al. CD97 stabilises the immunological synapse between dendritic cells and T cells and is targeted for degradation by the *Salmonella* effector SteD. PLoS Pathogens. 2021;**17**(7):e1009771

[52] Feasey NA, Dougan G, Kingsley RA. Invasive non-typhoidal *Salmonella* disease: An emerging and neglected tropical disease in Africa. Lancet. 2012;**379**(9835):2489-2499

[53] Bronzan RN, Taylor TE, Mwenechanya J, Tembo M, Kayira K, Bwanaisa L, et al. Bacteremia in Malawian children with severe malaria: Prevalence, etiology, HIV coinfection, and outcome. Journal of Infectious Diseases. 2007;**195**(6):895-904

[54] Takem EN, Roca A, Cunnington A. The association between malaria and nontyphoid *Salmonella* bacteraemia in children in sub-Saharan Africa: A literature review. Malaria Journal. 2014;**13**(1):1-13

[55] Mtove G, Amos B, Von Seidlein L, Hendriksen I, Mwambuli A, Kimera J, et al. Invasive salmonellosis among children admitted to a rural Tanzanian hospital and a comparison with previous studies. PLoS One. 2010;**5**(2):e9244

[56] Scott JAG, Berkley JA, Mwangi I, Ochola L, Uyoga S, MacHaria A, et al. Relation between falciparum malaria and bacteraemia in Kenyan children: A population-based, case-control study and a longitudinal study. The Lancet. 2011;**378**(9799):1316-1323

[57] Biggs HM, Lester R, Nadjm B, Mtove G, Todd JE, Kinabo GD, et al.

Invasive *Salmonella* infections in areas of high and low malaria transmission intensity in Tanzania. Clinical Infectious Diseases. 2014;**58**(5):638-647

[58] Nairz M, Schroll A, Demetz E, Tancevski I, Theurl I, Weiss G. "Ride on the ferrous wheel" - the cycle of iron in macrophages in health and disease. Immunobiology. 2015;**220**(2):280-294

[59] Gwamaka M, Kurtis JD, Sorensen BE, Holte S, Morrison R, Mutabingwa TK, et al. Iron deficiency protects against severe *Plasmodium falciparum* malaria and death in Young children. Clinical Infectious Diseases. 2012;**54**(8):1137-1144

[60] Abuga KM, Jones-Warner W, Hafalla JCR. Immune responses to malaria pre-erythrocytic stages: Implications for vaccine development. Parasite Immunology. 2021;**43**(2):e12795

[61] Mooney JP, DonVito SM, Jahateh M, Bittaye H, Keith M, Galloway LJ, et al. 'Bouncing back' from subclinical malaria: Inflammation and erythrocytosis after resolution of *P. falciparum* infection in Gambian children. Frontiers in Immunology. 2022;**13**:780525

[62] Taniguchi T, Miyauchi E, Nakamura S, Hirai M, Suzue K, Imai T, et al. *Plasmodium berghei* ANKA causes intestinal malaria associated with dysbiosis. Scientific Reports. 2015;**5**(1):1-13

[63] Chau JY, Tiffany CM, Nimishakavi S, Lawrence JA, Pakpour N, Mooney JP, et al. Malaria-associated L-arginine deficiency induces mast cell-associated disruption to intestinal barrier defenses against nontyphoidal *Salmonella* bacteremia. Infection and Immunity. 2013;**81**:3515-3526

[64] Walker GT, Yang G, Tsai JY, Rodriguez JL, English BC, Faber F, et al. Malaria parasite infection compromises colonization resistance to an enteric pathogen by reducing gastric acidity. Science Advances. 2021;**7**(27):eabd6232

[65] Brent AJ, Oundo JO, Mwangi I, Ochola L, Lowe B, Berkley JA. *Salmonella* bacteremia in Kenyan children. Pediatric Infectious Disease Journal. 2006;**25**(3):230-236

[66] Graham SM, Walsh AL, Molyneux EM, Phiri AJ, Molyneux ME. Clinical presentation of non-typhoidal *Salmonella* bacteraemia in Malawian children. Transactions of the Royal Society of Tropical Medicine and Hygiene. 2000;**94**(3):310-314

[67] Gordon MA, Banda HT, Gondwe M, Gordon SB, Boeree MJ, Walsh AL, et al. Non-typhoidal *Salmonella* bacteraemia among HIV-infected Malawian adults: High mortality and frequent recrudescence. AIDS. 2002;**16**(12):1633-1641

[68] Gordon MA. *Salmonella* infections in immunocompromised adults. Journal of Infection. 2008;**56**(6):413-422

[69] Février M, Dorgham K, Rebollo A. CD4 +T cell depletion in human immunodeficiency virus (HIV) infection: Role of apoptosis. Viruses. 2011;**3**(5):586-612

[70] Raffatellu M, Santos RL, Verhoeven DE, George MD, Wilson RP, Winter SE, et al. Simian immunodeficiency virus-induced mucosal interleukin-17 deficiency promotes *Salmonella* dissemination from the gut. Nature Medicine [Internet]. 2008;**14**(4):421-428. Available from: https://www.nature.com/articles/nm1743 [Accessed: June 18, 2025]

[71] Brenchley JM, Douek DC. Microbial translocation across the GI tract. Annual Review of Immunology. 2012;**30**:149-173

[72] Brenchley JM, Price DA, Schacker TW, Asher TE, Silvestri G, Rao S, et al. Microbial translocation is a cause of systemic immune activation in chronic HIV infection. Nature Medicine. 2006;**12**(12):1365-1371

[73] Moir S, Fauci AS. B cells in HIV infection and disease. Nature Reviews. Immunology. 2009;**9**(4):235-245

[74] MacLennan CA, Gilchrist JJ, Gordon MA, Cunningham AF, Cobbold M, Goodall M, et al. Dysregulated humoral immunity to nontyphoidal '*Salmonella*' in HIV-infected African adults. Science (1979). 2010;**328**(5977):508-512

[75] Owen SV, Wenner N, Canals R, Makumi A, Hammarlof DL, Gordon MA, et al. Characterization of the prophage repertoire of African *Salmonella typhimurium* ST313 reveals high levels of spontaneous induction of novel phage BTP1. Frontiers in Microbiology. 2017;**8**:235

[76] Ashton PM, Owen SV, Kaindama L, Rowe WPM, Lane CR, Larkin L, et al. Public health surveillance in the UK revolutionises our understanding of the invasive *Salmonella typhimurium* epidemic in Africa. Genome Medicine. 2017;**9**:92

[77] Herrero-Fresno A, Wallrodt I, Leekitcharoenphon P, Olsen JE, Aarestrup FM, Hendriksen RS. The role of the st313-td gene in virulence of *Salmonella typhimurium* ST313. PLoS One. 2014;**9**(1):e84566

[78] Kintz E, Davies MR, Hammarlof DL, Canals R, Hinton JC, Woude MW. A BTP1 prophage gene present in invasive non-typhoidal *Salmonella* determines composition and length of the O-antigen of the lipopolysaccharide. Molecular Microbiology. 2015;**96**(2):263-275

[79] Onsare RS, Micoli F, Lanzilao L, Alfini R, Okoro CK, Muigai AW, et al. Relationship between antibody susceptibility and lipopolysaccharide O-antigen characteristics of invasive and gastrointestinal nontyphoidal *Salmonellae* isolates from Kenya. PLoS Neglected Tropical Diseases. 2015;**9**(3):3573

[80] Hammarlöf DL, Kröger C, Owen SV, Canals R, Lacharme-Lora L, Wenner N, et al. Role of a single noncoding nucleotide in the evolution of an epidemic African clade of *Salmonella*. Proceedings of the National Academy of Sciences of the United States of America. 2018;**115**(11):2614-2623

[81] Faucher SP, Porwollik S, Dozois CM, McClelland M, Daigle F. Transcriptome of *Salmonella enterica* serovar Typhi within macrophages revealed through the selective capture of transcribed sequences. Proceedings of the National Academy of Sciences of the United States of America [Internet]. 2006;**103**:6. DOI: 10.1073/pnas.0509183103

[82] Canals R, Hammarlöf DL, Kröger C, Owen SV, Fong WY, Lacharme-Lora L, et al. Adding function to the genome of African *Salmonella typhimurium* ST313 strain D23580. PLoS Biology. 2019;**17**(1):e3000059

[83] Okoro CK, Barquist L, Connor TR, Harris SR, Clare S, Stevens MP, et al. Signatures of adaptation in human invasive *Salmonella typhimurium* ST313 populations from sub-Saharan Africa. PLoS Neglected Tropical Diseases. 2015;**9**(3):3611

[84] Lokken KL, Stull-Lane AR, Poels K, Tsolis RM. Malaria parasite-mediated alteration of macrophage function and

increased iron availability predispose to disseminated nontyphoidal *Salmonella* infection. Infection and Immunity. 2018;**86**(9):e00301-18

[85] Kingsley RA, Kay S, Connor T, Barquist L, Sait L, Holt KE, et al. Genome and transcriptome adaptation accompanying emergence of the definitive type 2 host-restricted *Salmonella enterica* Serovar Typhimurium pathovar. MBio. 2013;**4**(5). DOI: 10.1128/mbio.00565-13

[86] Parkhill J, Dougan G, James KD, Thomson NR, Pickard D, Wain J, et al. Complete genome sequence of a multiple drug resistant *Salmonella enterica* serovar Typhi CT18. Nature. 2001;**413**(6858):848-852

[87] McClelland M, Sanderson KE, Clifton SW, Latreille P, Porwollik S, Sabo A, et al. Comparison of genome degradation in Paratyphi A and Typhi, human-restricted serovars of *Salmonella enterica* that cause typhoid. Nature Genetics. 2004;**36**(12):1268-1274

[88] Liu WQ, Feng Y, Wang Y, Zou QH, Chen F, Guo JT, et al. *Salmonella paratyphi* C: Genetic divergence from *Salmonella choleraesuis* and pathogenic convergence with *Salmonella typhi*. PLoS One. 2009;**4**(2):e4510

[89] Thomson NR, Clayton DJ, Windhorst D, Vernikos G, Davidson S, Churcher C, et al. Comparative genome analysis of *Salmonella enteritidis* PT4 and *Salmonella gallinarum* 287/91 provides insights into evolutionary and host adaptation pathways. Genome Research. 2008;**18**(10):1624-1637

[90] Carden SE, Walker GT, Honeycutt J, Lugo K, Pham T, Jacobson A, et al. Pseudogenization of the secreted effector gene sseI confers rapid systemic dissemination of *S. typhimurium* ST313 within migratory dendritic cells. Cell Host & Microbe. 2017;**21**(2):182-194

[91] Carden S, Okoro C, Dougan G, Monack D. Non-typhoidal *Salmonella typhimurium* ST313 isolates that cause bacteremia in humans stimulate less inflammasome activation than ST19 isolates associated with gastroenteritis. Pathogens and Disease. 2015;**73**(4):23

[92] Chirwa EB, Dale H, Gordon MA, Ashton PM. What is the source of infections causing invasive nontyphoidal *Salmonella* disease? Open Forum Infectious Diseases. 2023;**10**:ofad086

[93] Kariuki S, Revathi G, Gakuya F, Yamo V, Muyodi J, Hart CA. Lack of clonal relationship between non-typhi *Salmonella* strain types from humans and those isolated from animals living in close contact. FEMS Immunology and Medical Microbiology. 2002;**33**(3):165-171

[94] Dione MM, Ikumapayi UN, Saha D, Mohammed NI, Geerts S, Ieven M, et al. Clonal differences between non-typhoidal *Salmonella* (NTS) recovered from children and animals living in close contact in the Gambia. PLoS Neglected Tropical Diseases. 2011;**5**(5):e1148

[95] Parsons BN, Humphrey S, Salisbury AM, Mikoleit J, Hinton JCD, Gordon MA, et al. Invasive non-typhoidal *Salmonella typhimurium* st313 are not host-restricted and have an invasive phenotype in experimentally infected chickens. PLoS Neglected Tropical Diseases. 2013;**7**(10):1-8

[96] Crump JA, Thomas KM, Benschop J, Knox MA, Wilkinson DA, Midwinter AC, et al. Investigating the meat pathway as a source of human nontyphoidal *Salmonella* bloodstream infections and diarrhea in East

Africa. Clinical Infectious Diseases. 2021;**73**(7):E1570-E1578

[97] Thye T, Krumkamp R, Lusingu JPA, Ofori LA, Minja DTR, Flieger A, et al. Non-typhoidal *Salmonella* transmission reservoirs in sub-Saharan Africa: A genomic assessment from a one health perspective. Antimicrobial Resistance and Infection Control. 2025;**14**(1):1-18

[98] Kumwenda B, Canals R, Predeus AV, Zhu X, Kröger C, Pulford C, et al. *Salmonella enterica* serovar Typhimurium ST313 sublineage 2.2 has emerged in Malawi with a characteristic gene expression signature and a fitness advantage. microLife. 2024;**5**:uqae005

[99] Van Puyvelde S, Pickard D, Vandelannoote K, Heinz E, Barbé B, de Block T, et al. An African *Salmonella typhimurium* st313 sublineage with extensive drug-resistance and signatures of host adaptation. Nature Communications. 2019;**10**(1):4280

[100] Ikhimiukor OO, Oaikhena AO, Afolayan AO, Fadeyi A, Kehinde A, Ogunleye VO, et al. Genomic characterization of invasive typhoidal and non-typhoidal *Salmonella* in southwestern Nigeria. PLoS Neglected Tropical Diseases. 2022;**16**(8):e0010716

[101] Yamba K, Kapesa C, Mpabalwani E, Hachaambwa L, Smith AM, Young AL, et al. Antimicrobial susceptibility and genomic profiling of *Salmonella enterica* from bloodstream infections at a tertiary referral hospital in Lusaka, Zambia, 2018-2019. IJID Regions. 2022;**3**:248-255

[102] Kanteh A, Sesay AK, Alikhan NF, Ikumapayi UN, Salaudeen R, Manneh J, et al. Invasive atypical non-typhoidal *Salmonella serovars* in the Gambia. Microbial Genomics. 2021;7(11):000677

[103] Mandomando I, MacEte E, Sigaúque B, Morais L, Quintó L, Sacarlal J, et al. Invasive non-typhoidal *Salmonella* in Mozambican children. Tropical Medicine and International Health. 2009;**14**(12):1467-1474

[104] Zhao J, Lu X, Tie A, Ngegba E, Wang L, Sun L, et al. Molecular diagnostics and next-generation sequencing reveal real etiological characteristics of invasive *Salmonella* infection in febrile illness in Freetown, Sierra Leone. Emerging Microbes & Infections. 2022;**11**(1):1416-1424

[105] Kalonji LM, Post A, Phoba MF, Falay D, Ngbonda D, Muyembe JJ, et al. Invasive *Salmonella* infections at multiple surveillance sites in the Democratic Republic of the Congo, 2011-2014. Clinical Infectious Diseases. 2015;**61**:S346-S353

[106] Pulford CV, Perez-Sepulveda BM, Canals R, Bevington JA, Bengtsson RJ, Wenner N, et al. Stepwise evolution of *Salmonella typhimurium* ST313 causing bloodstream infection in Africa. Nature Microbiology. 2020 [Internet];**6**(3):327-338. Available from: https://www.nature.com/articles/s41564-020-00836-1 [Accessed: March 4, 2024]

[107] Park SE, Pham DT, Pak GD, Panzner U, Maria Cruz Espinoza L, Von Kalckreuth V, et al. The genomic epidemiology of multi-drug resistant invasive non-typhoidal *Salmonella* in selected sub-Saharan African countries. BMJ Global Health. 2021;**6**(8):e005659

[108] Feasey NA, Masesa C, Jassi C, Faragher EB, Mallewa J, Mallewa M, et al. Three epidemics of invasive multidrug-resistant *Salmonella* bloodstream infection in Blantyre, Malawi, 1998-2014. Clinical Infectious Diseases. 2015;**61**(4):363-371

[109] Cassese D, Dimitri N, Breghi G. Spadafina T. Effectiveness of iNTS vaccination in sub-Saharan Africa. Scientific Reports [Internet]. 2025;**15**(1):3765. Available from: https://www.nature.com/articles/s41598-025-87659-4 [Accessed: May 31, 2025]

[110] Emary K, Bentsi-Enchill AD, Giersing BK, Gordon M, Dale H, Chirwa EB, et al. Landscape analysis of invasive non-typhoidal *Salmonella* (iNTS) disease and iNTS vaccine use case and demand: Report of a WHO expert consultation. Vaccine. 2025;**55**:127008

[111] Martin LB, Tack B, Marchello CS, Sikorski MJ, Owusu-Dabo E, Nyirenda T, et al. Vaccine value profile for invasive non-typhoidal *Salmonella* disease. Vaccine. 2024;**42**(19):S101-S124

[112] World Health Organization. Typhoid vaccines: WHO position paper, march 2018 – Recommendations. Vaccine [Internet]. 2019;**37**(2):214-216. Available from: https://www.sciencedirect.com/science/article/pii/S0264410X18304912 [Accessed: June 19, 2025]

[113] Tennant SM, Levine MM. Live attenuated vaccines for invasive *Salmonella* infections. Vaccine. 2015;**33**(Suppl 3):36-41

[114] Angelakopoulos H, Hohmann EL. Pilot study of phoP/phoQ-deleted *Salmonella enterica* serovar Typhimurium expressing *Helicobacter pylori* urease in adult volunteers. Infection and Immunity. 2000;**68**:2135-2141

[115] Hindle Z, Chatfield SN, Phillimore J, Bentley M, Johnson J, Cosgrove CA, et al. Characterization of *Salmonella enterica* derivatives harboring defined aroC and ssaV mutations by immunization of healthy volunteers. Infection and Immunity. 2002;**70**:3457-3467

[116] Ji HJ, Jang AY, Song JY, Ahn KB, Han SH, Bang SJ, et al. Development of live-attenuated *Salmonella typhimurium* vaccine strain using radiation mutation enhancement technology (R-MET). Frontiers in Immunology. 2022;**13**:931052

[117] Garcia P, Moscoso M, Fuentes-Valverde V, Rodicio MR, Herrera-Leon S, Bou G. A highly-safe live auxotrophic vaccine protecting against disease caused by non-typhoidal *Salmonella typhimurium* in mice. Journal of Microbiology, Immunology, and Infection. 2023;**56**:324-336

[118] Maryland U. *Salmonella* conjugates CVD 1000: Study of responses to vaccination with trivalent invasive *Salmonella* disease vaccine. 2021. Available from: https://clinicaltrials.gov/study/NCT03981952

[119] Maryland U. *Salmonella* conjugates CVD 2000: Study of responses to vaccination with trivalent *Salmonella* conjugate vaccine. 2022. Available from: https://clinicaltrials.gov/study/NCT05525546

[120] Tontini M, Berti F, Romano MR, Proietti D, Zambonelli C, Bottomley MJ, et al. Comparison of CRM197, diphtheria toxoid and tetanus toxoid as protein carriers for meningococcal glycoconjugate vaccines. Vaccine. 2013;**31**(42):4827-4833

[121] Shinefield HR. Overview of the development and current use of CRM197 conjugate vaccines for pediatric use. Vaccine. 2010;**28**(27):4335-4339

[122] Rondini S, Lanzilao L, Necchi F, O'Shaughnessy CM, Micoli F, Saul A, et al. Invasive African *Salmonella typhimurium* induces bactericidal antibodies against O-antigens. Microbial Pathogenesis. 2013;**63**:19-23

[123] Rondini S, Micoli F, Lanzilao L, Gavini M, Alfini R, Brandt C, et al. Design of glycoconjugate vaccines against invasive African *Salmonella enterica* serovar Typhimurium. Infection and Immunity. 2015;**83**(3):996-1007

[124] Micoli F, Rondini S, Alfini R, Lanzilao L, Necchi F, Negrea A. Comparative immunogenicity and efficacy of equivalent outer membrane vesicle and glycoconjugate vaccines against non-typhoidal *Salmonella*. Proc Natl Acad Sci USA. 2018;**115**(42):10428-10433

[125] Micoli F, Alfini R, Benedetto R, Necchi F, Schiavo F, Mancini F. GMMA is a versatile platform to design effective multivalent combination vaccines. Vaccines (Basel). 2020;**8**:540

[126] Hanumunthadu B, Kanji N, Owino N, Silva C, Robinson H, White R, et al. *Salmonella* vaccine study in oxford (SALVO) Trial TVOC. BMJ Open. 2023;**13**:72938

[127] Spadafina T. PEDVAC-iNTS starts a Phase 2 Clinical Trial of a Vaccine Against Invasive Non-Typhoidal Salmonellosis, iNTS-GMMA in Ghana [Internet]. 2024. Available from: https://pedvac-ints.eu/pedvac-ints-starts-a-phase-2-clinical-trial-of-a-vaccine-against-invasive-non-typhoidal-salmonellosis-ints-gmma-in-ghana/ [Accessed: June 19, 2025]

[128] Skidmore PD, Canals R, Ramasamy MN. The iNTS-GMMA vaccine: A promising step in non-typhoidal *Salmonella* vaccine development. Expert Review of Vaccines. 2023;**22**(9):918-920

[129] Malley R, Lu YJ, Sebastian S, Zhang F, Willer DO. Multiple antigen presenting system (MAPS): State of the art and potential applications. Expert Review of Vaccines. 2024;**23**:196-204

[130] Boerth EM, Gong J, Roffler B, Thompson CM, Song B, Malley SF, et al. Induction of broad immunity against invasive *Salmonella* disease by a quadrivalent combination *Salmonella* MAPS vaccine targeting *Salmonella enterica* serovars Typhimurium, Enteritidis, Typhi, and Paratyphi A. Vaccines (Basel). 2023;**11**:1671

Chapter 3

Salmonella and Public Health in Europe: The Role of Primary Care Physicians

Ana R. Miljković

Abstract

Salmonellosis remains one of the leading zoonotic diseases in Europe, with a significant impact on public health, health systems, and the economy. Despite prevention and control efforts, the incidence of infections caused by *Salmonella enteritidis* and *S. typhimurium serovars* has shown a tendency to stagnate in recent years. The chapter provides an overview of contemporary epidemiological trends in Europe, looking at regional differences, seasonal patterns, and the most common sources of infection. Particularly important is the recognition of vulnerable populations, such as children, the elderly, and the immunocompromised. Surveillance strategies implemented by national and European institutions are analyzed, with particular emphasis on the importance of the One Health approach in controlling the spread of diseases along the entire food chain. The role of primary care physicians has been recognized as crucial in the early detection of cases, patient education, and the implementation of prevention measures. Also, modern guidelines in the development of vaccines against non-typhoidal Salmonella are presented, as well as the need for multidisciplinary cooperation among health, veterinary, and sanitary institutions. Challenges such as antimicrobial resistance and insufficient cross-sectoral data sharing are highlighted. It concludes that for effective control of *salmonellosis*, it is necessary to improve public health policies, education, and biosecurity protocols while incorporating primary health care into broader prevention strategies. This is especially important in the modern context of climate change, global mobility, and the increased risk of multidrug-resistant strains.

Keywords: *salmonella* infections, zoonoses, public health, primary health care, food safety

1. Introduction

Salmonella is one of the most significant zoonotic pathogens globally [1], posing a continuous threat to public health due to its high incidence, widespread environmental presence, and ability to adapt to harsh conditions. Each year, *Salmonella* infections cause tens of millions of cases of gastroenteritis worldwide, with considerable morbidity and mortality. The European region, despite strong surveillance systems [2, 3], continues to face recurring outbreaks and increasing challenges such as antimicrobial resistance and emerging serovars.

This chapter explores the current public health impact of *salmonellosis* across Europe, emphasizing the pivotal role of primary care physicians in early detection, reporting, and public education. The discussion integrates epidemiological data, prevention strategies, and the importance of a One Health approach [2, 4] that bridges human, animal, and environmental health sectors. Special attention is given to regional surveillance systems, biosecurity measures in food production, and innovative directions in vaccine development [5, 6]. Through this multidisciplinary perspective, the chapter aims to highlight critical insights and practical solutions necessary for effective *salmonellosis* control in an era marked by globalization, climate change, and rising microbial resistance.

Salmonella spp. is one of the most important zoonotic pathogenic agents, causing an estimated 93.8 million cases of gastroenteritis worldwide annually, with 155,000 deaths. *Salmonella* is a gram-negative bacterium that uses flagella for locomotion. There are more than 2500 recognized serotypes. Salmonella is known to survive for a long time in foods with a low moisture content [1, 7]. *Salmonellosis* is considered a foodborne infection of the gastrointestinal tract that has been reported to have high incidence rates. The causative agent can pass from the feces of an infected person or animal to healthy ones. There are more than 2500 recognized serotypes [7].

Salmonellosis is a bacterial disease caused by non-typhoidal (*not S. Typhi and S. Paratyphi*), gram-negative bacilli of the genus *Salmonella*, causing gastroenteritis in humans. Infection usually occurs through eating contaminated food or water, as well as contact with another infected person or infected animal. Due to the high adaptability of *Salmonella* bacteria, they are widely distributed in the environment [8]. In Europe, salmonellosis remains one of the most commonly reported foodborne infections, with thousands of confirmed cases annually, as shown in the European Centre for Disease Prevention and Control (ECDC) Surveillance Atlas [9]. Although *salmonellosis* is mainly reported as a foodborne illness, it is estimated that about 10% of cases are due to direct contact with animals. *Salmonella* is a genus of highly diverse bacteria that live in the digestive tract of humans and animals. They are widely distributed in the environment thanks to their ability to survive and adapt even to extreme conditions. Among the more than 2600 *Salmonella* serovars described, clinical manifestations and mortality vary depending on the serovar and host characteristics (race, age, sex, diet, and/or immunity).

According to the World Health Organization (WHO), *Salmonella* is one of the four leading causes of diarrheal diseases worldwide. The processes of globalization contribute to the transmission of *salmonellosis*. In the U.S., up to 1.2 million cases of *salmonellosis* are reported each year. In European countries, the share of *salmonellosis* in the structure of food zoonoses is 30.2%. About half of the cases of *salmonellosis* are caused by *Salmonella enteritidis*, *typhimurium*, *newport*, and *javiana*. Chickens and pigs are considered to be the main reservoirs of salmonellosis [10].

2. Analysis of the public health significance of *salmonellosis* in Europe

2.1 Epidemiological data and trends

Each year, by the end of May, Member States of the European Union (EU) and the European Economic Area (EEA) are required to submit individual or aggregated data sets on zoonoses in humans in accordance with Directive 2003/99/EC. These data are submitted to the European surveillance system TESSy, analyzed, and forwarded to the European Food Safety Authority (EFSA) for the annual *European Union Zoonoses Report*. The report for 2021 includes data from 27 member states, Northern Ireland, and nine non-EU countries. According to the *Epidemiological Report 2021* by the European Centre for Disease Prevention and Control (ECDC), *salmonellosis* was the second most commonly reported zoonotic infection in the EU/EEA, with 620 reported outbreaks, 420 confirmed cases (an incidence of 16.6 per 100,000), and 73 recorded deaths [9].

After a decrease in cases during 2020 due to COVID-19 containment measures, 2021 saw an approximate 14% increase in cases. The highest rates were observed in children aged 0–4 years. Eggs remained the most common food source of infection, although outbreaks were also linked to contaminated wide areas, herbs, and seeds.

2.2 Country-specific reports

2.2.1 Poland and Bulgaria

In Poland, a study using the most recent epidemiological data reported 8294 cases of *salmonellosis* in 2021, corresponding to an incidence of 21.7 per 100,000 inhabitants. Compared to 2020, this represents an increase in case numbers, suggesting that the COVID-19 pandemic did not have a lasting impact on the incidence of *salmonellosis*. Interestingly, 2021 also marked the lowest percentage of hospitalizations for *salmonellosis* since 1998, possibly due to a shift toward outpatient management of milder cases [8].

In Bulgaria, national data show that salmonellosis continues to be a significant public health problem, with relatively high incidence rates despite year-to-year fluctuations. Diarrheal diseases caused by *Salmonella* bacteria remain prevalent, underscoring the need for continuous monitoring and prevention efforts [11].

2.2.2 Romania and Finland

A 2021 review by Romanian authors titled *"Salmonella as a Continuous Threat"* highlights that *Salmonella* infections remain a major public health concern worldwide. Despite existing control measures, the pathogen continues to cause numerous epidemics, including several recent outbreaks in Europe. The authors call for improved surveillance systems and prevention programs and emphasize the crucial role of primary care physicians in early case detection, public education, and timely reporting [12, 13].

In Finland, long-term surveillance between 1995 and 2022 revealed that about 60,000 *salmonellosis* cases were reported, with approximately 72% linked to international travel and only 18% domestically acquired. The COVID-19 pandemic led to a 74% reduction in international travel in 2020, mirrored by a 71% drop in *salmonellosis* cases, highlighting the strong link between travel and infection. This reinforces the preventive role of primary care physicians in advising patients on safe food and water consumption before travel and ensuring prompt reporting of symptoms upon return [13].

2.2.3 Netherlands and the role of travel

According to a 2021 report by the Dutch National Institute for Public Health and the Environment (RIVM), the number of laboratory-confirmed *salmonellosis* cases was 6 per 100,000 inhabitants, up slightly from 5 per 100,000 in 2020. In 2022, the estimated number of *salmonellosis* cases increased to 1290, compared to 1062 in 2021. *Salmonella enteritidis* remained the most frequent causative agent.

During the COVID-19 pandemic, the Netherlands experienced a marked reduction in salmonellosis incidence, particularly in travel-associated cases. This decline has been attributed to travel restrictions and the closure of catering establishments, both of which reduced exposure to contaminated food. These data further emphasize the public health relevance of travel-associated *salmonellosis* and the need for preventive strategies targeting travelers [14, 15].

3. Surveillance and prevention measures

3.1 Role of primary care physicians

According to the World Health Organization (WHO), *Salmonella* is one of the four leading causes of diarrheal disease globally and has the potential for severe domestic outcomes depending on age. It was emphasized that antibiotic-resistant strains are a growing problem—*Salmonella* is one of the microorganisms in which antimicrobial resistance is an important public health challenge. As a key prevention measure, the WHO recommends basic hygiene measures in food handling, especially thermal treatment of foodstuffs, which is a message that family medicine physicians should convey [3]. Due to the increase in antibiotic-resistant strains, as well as the significant morbidity, death, and economic burden that these infections cause, it is said that success lies in the development of vaccines against *typhoid* fever as well as a vaccine against *non-typhoidal Salmonella*, which could become an important tool in prevention in the future. For the time being, the role of primary care physicians remains in the implementation of hygiene measures and education of the population until these new tools are developed [5].

In order to prevent *salmonellosis*, in addition to the standard recommendations found in the guides of the Centers for Disease Control and Prevention, both for Europe and for regional centers in European countries, the role of general practitioners in the prevention of *salmonellosis* and early detection is crucial. General practitioners are often the first point of contact for patients with the health care system. Rapid recognition of symptoms of *salmonellosis* and timely referral to laboratory analyses (e.g., stool analysis, laboratory tests) allows for early detection of infection and prevention of further spread of the disease. Primary care physicians are also important in educating patients about proper hand hygiene, safe food handling, and the importance of heat treatment of food, which are essential measures in the prevention of *salmonellosis*. In many health systems of European countries, general practitioners are responsible for reporting confirmed cases of salmonellosis to the competent public health institutions, which allows the monitoring and control of epidemics, the so-called sentinel surveillance of infectious diseases. They are also the first to provide advice to particularly vulnerable groups, such as children, the elderly, and immunocompromised patients, on additional precautions to reduce the risk of infection. Primary care physicians (physicians for the adult population and pediatricians) can actively participate in health promotion and disease prevention campaigns, including the distribution of educational materials and the organization of community workshops at the local level in both health centers and local communities. Pediatricians also have a role to play in educating children about hygiene habits, and actions can be challenged in preschool and school institutions [2, 16, 17].

3.2 Food safety and hygiene control

In public catering and trading enterprises, where precautions for storing meat and eggs are often violated, such an intense infection of food products is a real fact. *Salmonella* reinoculation is most common in processing workshops of public catering facilities and shops [5, 7]. The problem of low-quality meat products and semi-finished products, especially associated with cooperative and private shops of small capacity. They are often housed in adapted rooms, insufficiently equipped, and insufficiently secured with containers, vehicles, warehouses, and refrigeration units. Employees, in most cases, have poor professional training. Many entrepreneurs process such meat into various sausages or smoked products or sell it in the form of semi-finished meat products, despite the fact that meat of forced slaughter, due to its limited suitability, is allowed to be used only for the manufacture of boiled sausages and canned food [5].

The latest scientific analysis of *salmonellosis* trends in Europe has shown that after years of decline, the incidence of infections caused by *Salmonella enteritidis* has stopped declining and stagnated in recent years. A group of authors from the Netherlands used a multi-criteria method to determine that the most likely cause of this stagnation is related to the level of primary poultry production (e.g., possible relaxation of control measures in some countries). It is proposed to intensify the improvement of the *Salmonella* control program in poultry farming and the One Health multidisciplinary cooperation of veterinarians, microbiologists, epidemiologists, and doctors in order to identify effective measures and reverse the trend back to decline. This implies that primary care physicians should work closely with public health authorities to monitor and report cases [14].

According to a report by the European Food Safety Authority and the European Centre for Disease Prevention and Control (ECDC) presenting the results of zoonotic monitoring and surveillance carried out in 2023 in the 27 Member States (MS), the United Kingdom (Northern Ireland), and 10 non-Member States, the two most commonly reported zoonoses in humans were *campylobacteriosis* and *salmonellosis*. *Salmonella enteritidis* has been the most commonly reported agent for reported foodborne cases and outbreaks. *Salmonella* in "eggs and egg products" was the causative agent/food of most concern. In 2023, this combination caused the highest number of outbreaks and cases of all food/cause combinations and was the second most hospitalized. *Salmonella* was also the cause associated with the majority of multicountry outbreaks reported in the EU in 2023 [2]. To protect consumers from *Salmonella*, the EU has adopted an integrated approach to food safety from farm to fork.

The approach consists of risk assessment and risk management measures involving all key actors: EU Member States, the European Commission, the European Parliament, EFSA, and the ECDC. All EU Member States have implemented improved *Salmonella* control programs in poultry, and risk managers have set targets to reduce *Salmonella* in poultry flocks (e.g., laying hens, broilers, turkeys). Prevention of *Salmonella* infection focuses on several categories, including sanitary control, caring for children with pets, and vaccination. Preventing *Salmonella* infection through good sanitation practices includes the supply of clean water and proper food handling. Contamination of water supplies can promote *Salmonella* infection, and chlorination with water purification is necessary to prevent infection. Food must be properly processed in kitchens. Persons handling food must implement good handwashing protocols. Street foods such as fruit and ice cream, along with animal products such as raw eggs, chicken, and uncooked meat, are important sources of infection [2, 4, 16].

3.3 Biosecurity in animal production

If we look at the transmission of infection from animal to human, we first look at the possibility that direct contact between domestic pigs and wild animals is one of the main routes of transmission of pathogens, especially in extensive farming systems such as open pens, rural households, and farms with access to forests, meadows, or neglected pastures. The risk is particularly pronounced in regions with large populations of wild boars.

The lack of adequate biosecurity measures, such as inadequate fencing, further increases the possibility of direct contact and transmission of diseases such as African swine fever (ASF), a transmissible viral disease that is most commonly spread through direct contact with infected animals. Pathogens can survive in the blood, tissue, and excreta of infected animals, allowing them to be transmitted during feeding or contact with contaminated surfaces. This complex mosaic of disease transmission points to the crucial need for strict biosecurity measures that include limiting contact with wildlife, using protective barriers (physical and sanitary), and controlling the presence of rodents and insects on farms, as well as constant monitoring of wild populations [12].

4. Future prevention measures: Develop vaccines

Invasive non-typhoidal *Salmonella enterica* serovars (NTS) are increasingly acquiring resistance to first-line antibiotics, so an effective vaccine would be a valuable tool in reducing morbidity and mortality from infection. Although vaccines against NTS for livestock are widely used, there are no licensed vaccines for use in humans [6]. The development of NTS vaccines involves candidates with live attenuated, subunit, and recombinant antigens. The development of a bivalent NTS vaccine would be necessary to protect against the dominant serovars *S. typhimurium* and *S. enteritidis*, or a multivalent vaccine that is combined with another enteric vaccine, such as the typhoid conjugate vaccine, for easier administration. Due to the lack of a controlled infection model for iNTS, field efficacy studies are needed, and interest in the development of a broadly protective *pan-Salmonella* vaccine was spurred by the 2021 WHO consultation on the strategy and preferred characteristics of these vaccines [18].

As part of more recent research in the field of *salmonellosis* prevention, authors from the *University of Florida* isolated 120 strains of *Salmonella* from wastewater in the Gainesville area and then tested the effectiveness of a vaccine that uses small extracellular vesicles (sEVs) as an antigen delivery system. The experimental model in mice showed a strong immune response without the need for the use of live bacteria, which is a potential advantage in terms of vaccine safety. Although the results are promising, further research is needed to examine the full potential of this approach in preventing netiphenoid salmonellosis [19].

The importance of such research is further confirmed by the findings of Makovska et al., who in a systematic review pointed to the role of wild animals and pests as important reservoirs of zoonotic pathogens, including *Salmonella spp.* In particular, the risks that arise from contact between domestic and wild animals in extensive breeding systems are singled out, which pose a challenge for biosecurity. This context further highlights the need for an integrated approach to prevention—through the development of vaccines, but also the implementation of biosecurity measures and the strengthening of cross-sectoral cooperation in line with the One Health concept [20].

5. Public health surveillance of *salmonellosis* in Serbia and the countries of the region

5.1 Intersectoral cooperation

In Serbia, salmonellosis is controlled within the system for reporting infectious diseases led by the Institute of Public Health "Dr Milan Jovanović Batut," in cooperation with the network of territorial institutes. The disease is compulsorily reported, and cases are recorded on the basis of clinical and laboratory criteria. According to available data, there has been a stable number of reports in the last 5 years, with the predominance of the *Salmonella enteritidis* serotype [21]. Surveillance is also carried out within the so-called sentinel networks, which enable the monitoring of trends and suspected outbreaks, especially in collective environments.

Countries in the region, such as Croatia, Bosnia and Herzegovina, and North Macedonia, apply similar principles in supervision, with certain differences in the capacities and organization of the system. In Croatia, the surveillance system is highly developed, and *salmonellosis* is regularly monitored through a network of microbiological laboratories and mandatory registration by a doctor. Seasonal peaks coincide with the summer months and increased consumption of animal foods [2]. A similar situation has been observed in Bosnia and Herzegovina, although there are challenges in terms of laboratory coverage and timely reporting.

In Bulgaria and Romania, according to national data, the incidence of salmonellosis remains high, despite the control measures implemented [11, 12]. The authors state that further improvement of the surveillance system and integration of the human and veterinary health sectors are necessary. In Finland, the majority of reported cases are travel-related, indicating the effectiveness of domestic control measures and the importance of counseling patients before travel [13].

Although national strategies in most countries are formally aligned with the European guidelines, their implementation in practice still varies. Insufficient integration between the public health, primary health care, and veterinary services, as well as the limited scope of laboratory testing, remains a challenge in the effective detection and control of infections [14]. In order to improve the public health response, it is recommended to develop standardized protocols for data exchange, strengthen laboratory capacities, and provide continuous education for health professionals—particularly primary care physicians, who are often the first point of contact for patients. The integration of these activities through the "One Health" approach is the basis for a sustainable and effective *salmonellosis* control system [2, 21].

5.2 Environmental and climate-related risks

Seasonal peaks coincide with the summer months and increased consumption of animal foods [2].

In Bulgaria and Romania, despite the control measures implemented, the incidence of *salmonellosis* remains high, which may also be influenced by environmental and infrastructural factors [11, 12].

Although not explicitly detailed in the provided paragraph, environmental and climate-related risks such as higher ambient temperatures, poor infrastructure, inadequate food storage, and the presence of vectors (like flies or rodents) are implied contributors to seasonal variation and regional challenges in controlling *salmonellosis.*

6. One health approach in *salmonellosis* control

6.1 Institutional frameworks and reporting systems

The concept of One Health is based on the understanding that human, animal, and environmental health are inextricably linked. Zoonoses, such as *salmonellosis*, are of enormous importance for the development of effective prevention and control strategies. The One Health approach involves coordinated collaboration between health professionals, veterinarians, microbiologists, epidemiologists, environmentalists, and food safety experts. *Salmonella* is a classic example of a foodborne pathogen that originates in domestic and wild animals, most commonly poultry and pigs. In the European Union, a number of *salmonellosis* outbreaks have been linked to contaminated eggs, meat, or processed products. Therefore, the management of this pathogen cannot be reduced exclusively to the clinical level but requires supervision of the entire food chain—from farm to table [2, 4].

In the fight against *salmonellosis*, veterinary medicine plays a role in the supervision of animals and the implementation of biosecurity measures on farms, as well as in the vaccination of livestock against certain serotypes. On the other hand, human medicine, especially at the primary health care level, is responsible for early identification of infections, reporting cases, and educating the population about the risks until a vaccine against *Salmonella* is developed as the strategically most important form of prevention [5, 18].

Reports by EFSA and ECDC state that countries that have implemented the One Health approach (e.g., the Netherlands, Sweden, and Finland) have achieved significant reductions in the number of *salmonellosis* cases thanks to joint surveillance programs, data sharing, and standardized protocols [2, 14]. Although the One Health concept also exists in the public health strategies of the Republic of Serbia, its practical application is still limited. It is necessary to strengthen institutional cooperation, develop integrated information systems, and include primary care physicians in the wider public health network [21].

6.2 Regional challenges and integration

Climate change, water and soil pollution, and inadequate disposal of wastewater and farm waste increase the risk of spreading *Salmonella*. The environmental aspect of the disease is often overlooked, although it is known that *Salmonella* can survive in water and soil and thus indirectly threaten the human population [20].

For the successful control of *salmonellosis* in the modern context of global trends and climate change, it is necessary to establish a national One Health Council [2, 14], strengthen laboratory capacities, and educate primary care physicians, who are currently the most important for early recognition and primary prevention. It is also necessary to develop protocols for data exchange and continuously invest in biosecurity in animal husbandry. The One Health approach is a sustainable solution that, through integrated intersectoral cooperation for human, animal, and environmental health, can contribute to reducing the incidence of diseases, responding to epidemics in a timely manner, and making more efficient use of available resources [6, 14].

7. Conclusion

Despite advances in surveillance, prevention, and education of the population, *salmonellosis* remains a serious public health challenge in Europe. Epidemiological data indicate stagnation in reducing incidence, the emergence of new serovars, and the increasing frequency of multidrug-resistant strains, which further complicates the treatment and control of the disease. Effectively combating *salmonellosis* requires a coordinated, multidisciplinary approach involving the health system, veterinary services, the food industry, and public health institutions. The role of primary care physicians is particularly important—both in the early recognition and reporting of cases, as well as in the continuous education of patients on hygiene measures and safe food handling.

The implementation of the One Health approach, the strengthening of laboratory capacities, the improvement of biosecurity measures in animal husbandry, the development of protocols for data exchange between sectors, and the development of a vaccine for human use are key steps toward a sustainable strategy for the control of this zoonosis in the modern context of global trends, climate change, and antimicrobial resistance.

8. Conclusions

This chapter is part of a broader effort to enhance understanding of zoonotic diseases in Europe, highlighting the importance of a multidisciplinary approach in public health.

Acknowledgements

The author also wishes to acknowledge the support and collaboration of colleagues and public health institutions whose insights and shared data contributed to the quality of this work. No external funding was received for the preparation of this manuscript.

Conflict of interest

The author declares no conflict of interest.

Notes/thanks/other declarations

I would like to express my sincere gratitude for the opportunity to be part of the group of authors selected to contribute to this chapter. I am especially thankful that my capabilities were recognized and that I was entrusted with the responsibility to develop and write this work.

Acronyms and abbreviations

ASF	African swine fever
CDC	Centers for Disease Control and Prevention
COP	coefficient of performance
ECDC	European Centre for Disease Prevention and Control
EFSA	European Food Safety Authority
EU	European Union
FAO	Food and Agriculture Organization
FL	Florida
GMMA	Generalized Modules for Membrane Antigens
iNTS	invasive non-typhoidal *Salmonella*
MS	member states
NTS	non-typhoidal serovars *Salmonellae*
PCPs	primary care physicians
RIVM	National Institute of Public Health and the Environment (Netherlands)
SALVO	*Salmonella* vaccine study in Oxford
sEVs	small extracellular vesicles
TESSy	The European Surveillance System
U.S.	United States
WHO	World Health Organization

Author details

Ana R. Miljković
Faculty of Medicine, Department of General Medicine and Geriatrics, University of Novi Sad, Novi Sad, Serbia

*Address all correspondence to: ana.miljkovic@mf.uns.ac.rs

References

[1] Galán-Relaño Á, Valero-Díaz A, Huerta-Lorenzo B, Gómez-Gascón L, Mena-Rodríguez MÁ, Carrasco-Jiménez E, et al. Salmonella and salmonellosis: An update on public health implications and control strategies. Animals. 2023;**13**(23):3666. DOI: 10.3390/ani13233666

[2] European Food Safety Authority (EFSA) and European Centre for Disease Prevention and Control (ECDC). The European Union one health 2023 zoonoses report. EFSA Journal. 2024;**22**(12):9106. DOI: 10.2903/j.efsa.2024.9106

[3] World Health Organization (WHO). Salmonella (Non-Typhoidal). Geneva: WHO; 2023. Available from: https://www.who.int/news-room/fact-sheets [Accessed: August 9, 2025]

[4] European Food Safety Authority (EFSA). Salmonella. Parma: EFSA; 2025. Available from: https://www.efsa.europa.eu/en/topics/topic/salmonella [Accessed: August 9, 2025]

[5] Micoli F, Mancini F, Pezzicoli A, Launay O, Rossi O, Buccato S, et al. GMMA is a versatile platform to design effective multivalent combination vaccines. Vaccine. 2020;**8**(3):540. DOI: 10.3390/vaccines8030540

[6] World Health Organization (WHO). Nontyphoidal Salmonella Disease. Geneva: WHO; 2025. Available from: https://www.who.int [Accessed: August 9, 2025]. (See Sections: Surveillance and Reporting; Food Safety and Biosecurity; Vaccine Research and Development)

[7] Ehuwa O, Jaiswal AK, Jaiswal S. Salmonella, food safety and food handling practices. Food. 2021;**10**(5):907. Available from: https://www.mdpi.com/2304-8158/10/5/907 [Accessed: August 9, 2025]

[8] Milczarek M, Czarkowski MP, Sadkowska-Todys M. Salmonellosis in Poland in 2021. Przegląd Epidemiologiczny. 2023;**77**(4):504-519. DOI: 10.32394/pe.77.41. [Language: Polish]

[9] European Centre for Disease Prevention and Control (ECDC). Surveillance Atlas of Infectious Diseases – Salmonellosis. Stockholm: ECDC; 2022. Available from: https://atlas.ecdc.europa.eu [Accessed: August 9, 2025]

[10] Podavalenko A, Malysh N, Zadorozhna V, Chemych M, Biryukova S, Chorna I. Incidence and risk factors of salmonellosis in Ukraine. Folia Medica Cracoviensia. 2021;**61**(2):91-102. DOI: 10.24425/fmc.2021.137226

[11] Pavlova M, Stoyanova R. Analysis of diarrheal diseases in humans caused by Salmonella in Bulgaria. Bulgarian One Health Journal. 2024:114-125. Available from: https://www.onehealthjournal.eu/articles/public-health/analysis-of-diarrheal-diseases-in-humans-caused-by-salmonella-in-bulgaria

[12] Popa GL, Papa MI. Salmonella spp. infection – A continuous threat worldwide. Germs. 2021;**11**(1):88-96. DOI: 10.18683/germs.2021.1244

[13] Suominen K, Ollgren J, Leinonen E, Rimhanen-Finne R. Reporting of salmonellosis markedly declined in Finland during 28 years of surveillance, 1995-2022. Microorganisms. 2025;**13**(3):693. DOI: 10.3390/microorganisms13030693

[14] Mughini-Gras L, van Pelt W, Franz E, Friesema IHM, Pijnacker R, van den

Bunt G, et al. Impact of the COVID-19 pandemic on human salmonellosis in the Netherlands. Epidemiology and Infection. 2021;**149**:e254. DOI: 10.1017/S0950268821002557

[15] Benincà E, Pijnacker R, Friesema IHM, Kretzschmar M, Franz E, Mughini-Gras L. Disease Burden of Food-Related Pathogens in the Netherlands, 2021. Bilthoven: RIVM; 2022. Report No. 2022-0173

[16] Ajmera A, Shabbir N. Salmonella. In: StatPearls [Internet]. Treasure Island (FL): StatPearls Publishing; 2025. Available from: https://www.statpearls.com [Accessed: August 9, 2025]. (See section: Epidemiology)

[17] Klochko A, Bronze MS. Salmonella Infection (Salmonellosis) Treatment & Management. Medscape; 2023. Available from: https://emedicine.medscape.com/article/228174-treatment [Accessed: August 9, 2025]

[18] Hanumunthadu B, Kanji N, Owino N, et al. Salmonella vaccine study in Oxford (SALVO) trial: Protocol for an observer-participant blind randomised placebo-controlled trial of the iNTS-GMMA vaccine. BMJ Open. 2023;**13**(11):e072938. DOI: 10.1136/bmjopen-2023-072938

[19] Emerson LE, Bhimani S, Rainey AL, Maurelli AT, Ferraro MJ. Evaluating small extracellular vesicle-based vaccination across heterologous Salmonella strains isolated from wastewater. Infection and Immunity. 2025;**93**(2):e00485-e00424. DOI: 10.1128/iai.00485-24

[20] Makovska I, Podgórska I, Škoda J, Grądzka M, Kowalczyk A, Kołodziej J, et al. The role of wildlife and pests in the transmission of pathogenic agents to domestic pigs: A systematic review. Animals. 2023;**13**(11):1830. DOI: 10.3390/ani13111830

[21] Ministry of Health of the Republic of Serbia. Public Health Strategy of the Republic of Serbia 2018-2026. Belgrade: Ministry of Health; 2018. Available from: https://www.pravno-informacioni-sistem.rs [Accessed: August 9, 2025]. [Language: Serbian]

Section 2

Mechanisms of Transmission, Dissemination, Virulence and Antimicrobial Resistance

Chapter 4

The Role of Poultry Food Matrices in Transmitting *Salmonella*

Greeshma Bharathan and Shabarinath Srikumar

Abstract

Salmonella spp. continues to represent a leading cause of foodborne illness worldwide, with poultry products serving as a significant reservoir and vehicle for human infection. This chapter provides a comprehensive analysis of the role of poultry matrices in the transmission dynamics of *Salmonella*, beginning with the pathogen's biology, virulence mechanisms, and environmental adaptability. Diverse poultry matrices—including raw cuts, marinated products, vacuum-packed items, frozen preparations, and ready-to-eat formulations—are examined for their unique physicochemical properties and the influence these exert on *Salmonella* survival, colonization, and growth kinetics. Detection methodologies, including traditional culture-based approaches and advanced molecular techniques, are evaluated for their applicability in complex food matrices. In addition, the chapter reviews key epidemiological trends, notable serotypes linked to poultry-associated outbreaks, and the implications of antimicrobial resistance. Integrated control strategies, regulatory frameworks, and consumer-level interventions are also discussed. Collectively, the chapter highlights the need for matrix-specific risk assessment models and targeted mitigation strategies to more effectively control *Salmonella* across the poultry supply chain.

Keywords: *Salmonella*, foodborne illness, poultry matrices, regulatory framework, control strategies

1. Introduction

Non-typhoidal *Salmonella* (NTS) is the primary causative agent of foodborne infections worldwide. They are widely distributed in nature, with over 2500 serotypes based on their differences in the lipopolysaccharide (O antigen) and flagellar antigens (H antigens) [1]. The most common serotype is *Salmonella enterica* subspecies *enterica*, which causes almost 99% of human and animal infections. This serotype is further divided into Typhoidal and Non-typhoidal serovars. The typhoidal serovars include the Typhi, Sendai, and Paratyphi A, B, and C, which are common in developing countries with poor sanitation [2]. Non-typhoidal serovars, such as *S.* Typhimurium and *S.* Enteritidis, infect a broad range of warm-blooded animals, including humans. Some serotypes are host-specific, including *S.* Gallinarum, which infects poultry, and *S.* Dublin, which infects cattle [3].

2. Historical perspective of the organism

Salmonella belongs to the Gram-negative, facultative anaerobes, non-spore-forming rods that are motile with peritrichous flagella. They are the core group of the Enterobacteriaceae family and are thought to have originated 160–180 million years ago from the same ancestor as *Escherichia coli*, with *E. coli* and some *Salmonella* serovars adapting to mammals and other *Salmonella* serovars adapting to reptiles. *Salmonella enterica* and *Salmonella bongori* are the only two species of the genus *Salmonella*, according to the Centre for Disease Control and Prevention. Even though there are only two species of *Salmonella* known to science, their importance should not be undervalued because *S. enterica* has approximately 2500 serovars and six subspecies [4].

Salmonella was named after D.E. Salmon, whose lab (bacteriologist Theobald Smith) isolated the *S.* Cholerasuis from the porcine intestine. The first report of a foodborne salmonellosis outbreak dates to 1888, when 58 persons from 25 different families developed acute gastroenteritis after eating beef. Gartner isolated the infectious agent from the infected cow (from which the beef was taken) and its organs. The organism was called "Gartner bacillus," which was later identified to be serotype Enteritidis, according to Kaufmann serotyping [5].

As per the degree of host restriction [6], *Salmonella* serovars are categorized into the following:

- *Host-restricted serovars*, which can infect a single host species and induce an illness akin to typhoid. *S.* Gallinarum and *S.* Pullorum in poultry and *S.* Typhi, *S.* Sendai, and *S.* Paratyphi A, B, and C in humans are examples of this group.

- *Host-adapted serovars* are pathogens that are linked to a particular host species but can infect different hosts. This category includes *Salmonella* Typhisuis and *S.* Choleraesuis.

- *Broad-host-range serovars*, which can colonize the digestive tract of a variety of animals but never cause systemic infections. Most of the serovars in this group, the most prevalent strains of which are *S.* Typhimurium and *S.* Enteritidis, are collectively referred to as non-typhoidal serovars (NTS).

Salmonella is one of the most frequently isolated pathogens from foodborne outbreaks across the world. It contributes to a huge financial burden in the form of surveillance, prevention, and treatment of disease in developed as well as underdeveloped countries. Since they are so versatile, *Salmonella* can live in a variety of environmental niches, including those found in meat and animal products. This ecological success is partly attributed to an intricate physiology that allows for resilience to various environmental pressures and the utilization of a variety of nutritional sources. *Salmonella* employs a complex virulence strategy that allows it to survive in the immune systems and the guts of many different animals, including humans. Therefore, to regulate the pathogen's levels throughout the food production chain, a variety of strategies are being researched and developed [7].

3. Biology and pathogenicity of *Salmonella*

3.1 Pathogenesis of the disease

Salmonella infection occurs through the ingestion of contaminated food or water. On entering the stomach, *Salmonella* encounters a highly acidic pH (pH 2), which is overcome by maintaining the pH-homeostatic function as part of the acid-tolerant response of *Salmonella* [8]. This helps to maintain a higher intracellular pH than that of the external environment. On reaching the small intestine, *Salmonella* has to overcome the intestinal mucus layer to adhere and attach themselves to the intestinal epithelial cells [9]. Studies in mice have shown that *Salmonella* gains entry into the intestinal epithelium through the M cells of Peyer's patches [10]. As an alternative, the dendritic cells that line the intestinal lumen can directly take up bacteria through their dendrites and open the tight junctions of the intestinal epithelium [11].

3.2 Attachment and mechanism of dissemination of *Salmonella*

Attachment to the host cell is the foremost and key step in the pathogenesis of the bacterium. This is enabled by the specific binding of protein structures (Adhesins) that are present on the surface of the bacterium to different receptors on the host cell [12]. These adhesins bind to polyhydroxylated glycan or glycosaminoglycans (GAGs) on the host cell surface [13–15].

Salmonella has well-developed fimbrial adhesins that aid in attaching itself to the host cell. Fimbriae are non-flagellar, filamentous, extracellular appendages with 0.5–10 μm length and 2–8 nm width. They are typically involved in adhesion and many other functions, including interaction with macrophages, biofilm formation, intestinal persistence, and bacterial aggregation [16].

Salmonella fimbriae aid in invading non-phagocytic enterocytes in the intestinal epithelium and subsequently adhere to the epithelium [17]. They interact with several receptors on the host cell and play an important role in *Salmonella* pathogenesis [18]. The fimbriae are divided into three different categories based on their assembly: CU, N/P, and T4 fimbriae. Members of the type 1 fimbriae family are called *fim* fimbriae. They are distinguished by their ability to attach to host cells and exhibit mannose-sensitive hemagglutination. The adhesion to the host cell receptor is a characteristic feature of *fim*H, which is found at the tip of *fim* fimbriae. The most researched FimH, which the *fim* operon encodes, is a bi-domain protein that is extremely specific to residues of mannose. While the other N-terminal domain binds to host receptors, the C-terminal domain is utilized to integrate FimH into the organelle [19]. A variety of factors, including low temperature, low osmolarity, and restricted nutrition, influence curli fimbriae assembly and expression. Different extracellular matrix proteins, such as laminin, fibronectin, and fibrinogen, may facilitate curli fimbriae's adhesion to host cells. It is suggested that curli fimbriae interact with numerous host proteins to promote bacterial growth within the host. Plasminogen, activated from a proenzyme form, breaks down fibrin and soft tissues. Plasmin is activated because of curli fimbriae attaching to plasminogen. Because plasmin breaks down soft tissue, it may provide an opportunity for bacteria to enter the host cell [20].

Apart from these fimbrial adhesins, *Salmonella* also possesses non-fimbrial adhesins which aid in the attachment of the pathogen to the intestinal epithelial cells.

a. SiiE: It is a non-fimbrial adhesin protein that helps in attachment to the host cell. This is encoded by SPI-4. It is composed of three subunits: SiiF, which acts as the inner membrane and has ATPase activity, SiiD, which is the transmembrane unit, and SiiC, which acts as the outer membrane unit.

b. Biofilm association protein (BapA): It is important in biofilm formation. This is secreted through T1SS and exists on the surface of the bacteria. It is regulated by the CsgD regulator.

c. Resistance to Complement killing (Rck): It is an outer membrane protein that plays an important role in invading the host cell. Rck mediates complement resistance by inhibiting the polymerization of C9 on the bacterial surface. Rck attaches itself to the Epidermal Growth Factor Receptor (EGFR) which leads to the autophosphorylation of the EGFR cytosolic tail. This signal activates Src, which aids in bacterial internalization.

d. PhoP-activated gene N (PagN): The outer membrane protein PagN binds to the heparan sulfate receptor on the eukaryotic host cell. Inside a macrophage, under cation-limiting conditions, PhoP activates PagN.

e. *Salmonella* Typhi Invasion (STIV): This protein plays a prominent role in the systemic spread and colonization of the intestine during infection of *S.* Typhi. STIV attaches to Met, which is the tyrosine kinase of the intestinal host cell. This leads to the phosphorylation of Met, which results in the polymerization of actin filaments and the engulfment of the bacteria.

f. MisL: Encoded by SPI-3, this outer membrane protein binds to fibronectin. This enables *Salmonella* to invade and persist in the intestinal epithelium.

3.3 Entry into the host cell

Salmonella is mainly transmitted by the consumption of contaminated food or water. A large bacterial load in the food or the buffering capacity of the food can help the pathogen evade the acidity of the stomach. The pathogen then travels down the intestinal tract to reach the large intestine. With the help of adhesins, flagella, and chemotactic systems, the bacterium reaches close to the intestinal epithelium, which leads to the activation of Type 3 Secretion System (T3SS) encoded by *Salmonella* Pathogenicity Island-1 (SPI-1). This attachment delivers several effector proteins into the host cell to modulate various host responses [21].

In the case of *Salmonella* infections, the host's inflammatory response is critical for the pathogen to colonize the intestinal tract. This response aids in the internalization of the bacteria and alteration of the transcriptional profile of the host-infected cell, which leads to inflammation. The effector proteins SopE, SopE2, and SopB lead to the activation of Rho-family GTPases, which leads to the rearrangement of the actin cytoskeleton and the internalization of the bacteria into the *Salmonella*-containing vacuole. Once internalized, intracellular environments like low pH and low magnesium concentrations lead to the activation of the T3SS encoded by SPI-2, which allows the bacteria to avoid innate immune mechanisms and replicate in the host cell. The infected cell produces proinflammatory cytokines like interleukin-8 (IL-8), tumor necrosis factor (TNF), and IL-1β,

DOI: http://dx.doi.org/10.5772/intechopen.1012025

which in turn allow for the recruitment of other immune cells like macrophages and neutrophils. This alters the lumen environment of the intestine and leads to an increase in antimicrobial peptides, which can deplete the normal resident microflora of the gut. These inflamed tissues also provide nutrients and electron acceptors that are required for the multiplication of *Salmonella* in the lumen of the intestine [22, 23].

3.4 Survival in intestinal epithelial cells

To survive inside the epithelial cell (M-cell), *Salmonella* has to escape the action of lysosomal enzymes. This is achieved by preventing the fusion with lysosomes. When inside the vacuole, *Salmonella* activates the *de novo* formation of the F-actin network of mesh around the vacuoles, called vacuole-associated actin polymerization (VAP). Then the SCVs move to a perinuclear position, close to the Golgi apparatus, to obtain nutrients. This enables the replication of the bacteria inside the vacuole. Moreover, intracellular *Salmonella* also induces the formation of long filamentous membrane structures called *Salmonella-induced* Filaments (SIFs). They are tubular aggregates that originate from SCVs and extend through the host cell, which provides increased nutrients for the bacteria in the vacuole. The vacuole then moves to the basolateral membrane and releases the internal bacterial cells into the submucosa, which are then internalized by phagocytes, including neutrophils, inflammatory monocytes that differentiate into macrophages, and dendritic cells (a type of macrophage that functions as an antigen-presenting cell). The bacterial cells that have traversed the intestinal epithelium through the M-cell reach the Peyer's patches and mesenteric lymph nodes through the intestinal lymph. Once phagocytosed by macrophages, *Salmonella* activates a similar phenomenon in phagocytes and survives and replicates inside a vacuole. These phagocytes then migrate through the bloodstream to spread the bacterium to tissues like the spleen and liver, where the bacteria replicate and cause infection [24].

3.5 Effector proteins involved in various stages of *Salmonella* pathogenesis

Once *Salmonella* has attached to the intestinal epithelium, T3SS-1 gets activated, which injects several effector proteins into the host cell to trigger the bacterial engulfment and proinflammatory response, which leads to the infection. The activation of T3SS-1 requires the protein DsbA, which is a disulfide oxidoreductase that forms periplasmic disulfide bonds to enable proper folding and assembly of proteins. The effector proteins SopE, SopE2, and SopB activate CDC 42, which leads to the formation of a signaling complex that includes p21-activated kinase (PAK1), transforming growth factor β-activating kinase-1 (TAK1), and tumor necrosis factor (TNF)-associated factor-6 (TRAF6). This in turn, activates nuclear factor-κB (NF-κB) and proinflammatory cytokine production. SopA effector protein, which is an E3 ubiquitin ligase, ubiquitylates the regulators TRIM56 and TRIM65, thereby activating the retinoic acid-inducible gene I protein (RIG-I) and melanoma differentiation-associated protein 5 (MDA5) signaling pathway to enable inflammation of the host cell. The SPI-1 effector protein SopD acts as a GTPase-activating protein (GAP) for RAB8 and stimulates inflammation by inhibiting the activity of RAB8. These responses activate the cytoskeletal remodeling and induction of the proinflammatory responses [21].

3.6 Downregulation of inflammation

The internalization of the bacteria and the proinflammatory responses will lead to damage to the intestinal epithelial cells, which enables the bacteria to get the required nutrients for their survival and multiplication. However, overactivation of these responses can alter the equilibrium (homeostasis) of the host cell, which can interfere with the replication of *Salmonella*. To overcome this, *Salmonella* has mechanisms to downregulate these inflammatory responses with the help of the following anti-inflammatory effector molecules [21].

- SptP—GTPase-activating protein for CDC42 and disrupts the actin cytoskeleton formation.

- PipA, GtgA, and GogA—Proteolytically cleave the NF-κB transcription factors RelA and RelB.

- SseK1 and SseK2—inhibit NF-κB signaling pathway by the transfer of N-acetylglucosamine to proteins.

- AvrA—acetylates MKK4 and MKK7 (mitogen-activated protein kinase) and blocks the signaling pathway.

- SpvC—phosphothreonine lyase which targets MAPKs, extracellular signal-regulated kinase 1 (ERK1), ERK2, and p38. This leads to decreased expression of proinflammatory cytokines like IL-8 and TNF-α and reduces neutrophil infiltration at the site of infection.

- SopB—phosphoinositide phosphatase activates phosphoinositide-3-kinase (PI3K) dependent signaling pathway.

- SopD—removes RAB8 from GDP-dissociation inhibitor (GDI).

- GogC—activates transcription of STAT-dependent signaling and anti-inflammatory cytokines like IL-10.

- Degradation of ubiquitylated TRIM56 and TRIM 65.

3.7 Competition with normal gut microflora

Salmonella-induced host response alters the composition of intestinal microbiota, suppressing its growth and offering an advantage for the growth of *Salmonella*. Large amounts of hydrogen sulfide produced by colonic bacteria react with reactive oxygen species and thiosulfate to produce tetrathionate. This tetrathionate can be used as an electron acceptor by *Salmonella* due to the presence of *ttr* genes located in SPI-2. This allows *Salmonella* to survive in the anaerobic environment of the intestinal mucosa. Moreover, SopE also induces the expression of nitric oxide synthase to produce nitric oxide (produced in activated macrophages), which reacts with reactive oxygen species (ROS) to form nitrate. Nitrate can also be utilized as an anaerobic electron acceptor by *Salmonella* [9].

4. Poultry food matrices

4.1 Definition and characteristics

The edible part of any domesticated bird, including chicken, duck, turkey, goose, guinea fowl, and Japanese quail, is referred to as poultry meat. The demand for high-quality animal protein and food security is met in large part by poultry meat. Because of the increased demand for poultry meat, global poultry production has been steadily increasing [25]. The term "*poultry product*" is defined as poultry that has been slaughtered for human consumption, with the removal of blood, feathers, feet, head, and viscera conducted following regulations established by the Secretary of Agriculture. It also includes any edible portion of poultry, as well as any food product intended for human consumption that contains such edible portions, either as a standalone component or in combination with other ingredients, unless specifically exempted by the Secretary [26].

The consumption of poultry meat has increased in recent decades which could be due to the following reasons: (1) The nutritional content of poultry products (rich protein content, reduced fat and cholesterol content), (2) Their processing suitability facilitates the development of value-added meat products that are more appealing, convenient, and user-friendly for consumers, (3) lower price compared to other meats like red meat [27]. Compared to other types of meat, poultry is more suitable for processing due to its neutral flavor, uniform and desirable texture, and light coloration. These attributes enable manufacturers to tailor flavor profiles (e.g., spicy or mild) and textures to meet specific market demands and target consumer groups (e.g., adults or children) [28]. Chicken contributes approximately 13.9% to the total animal protein intake and 7.2% to the overall protein consumption in the United States. In comparison, turkey, duck, and other poultry species collectively account for only 0.2% of animal protein and 0.1% of total protein intake [29].

Poultry production involves several stages before products reach consumers. For broilers, the process starts with raising chicks and continues through processing to produce a range of consumable products and by-products [30]. The US poultry industry operates under a vertically integrated system that includes hatcheries, feed mills, breeders, broiler farms, processing facilities, and distribution networks [31]. This model promotes efficiency and maintains quality control throughout the supply chain [32]. The proportion of poultry meat in total global meat production rose significantly from 8.3% in 1985 to 26.57% in 2021, reflecting the rapid expansion of the poultry industry. Despite this growth, the intensification of modern poultry farming systems has introduced a range of complex factors that influence both production and processing. These complexities present challenges in consistently ensuring the production of high-quality poultry meat for the market. Hence, it becomes necessary that we ensure the microbial safety of poultry meat products in the context of increasing consumption and production [33].

4.2 Physicochemical properties relevant to *Salmonella* survival

The high nutrient density of poultry products supports the proliferation of various microorganisms, leading to spoilage and potential foodborne illness. Microbial growth in livestock-derived foods is influenced by numerous factors, both inherent to the product and related to its storage environment. These influences are generally categorized into intrinsic and extrinsic factors. Intrinsic factors are those inherent to the food itself and include nutrient composition, water activity, pH, oxidation-reduction potential, natural biological barriers, antimicrobial compounds, and the presence of competitive microflora. Extrinsic factors pertain to the external conditions during storage, such as temperature, relative humidity, and the type and concentration of surrounding gases. A comprehensive understanding of these factors and their interactions is essential for developing effective strategies to inhibit the growth of spoilage organisms and foodborne pathogens [34].

5. Sources and routes of contamination in poultry

5.1 Breeders and hatchery

Salmonella can enter poultry production systems through multiple routes and spread *via* both vertical and horizontal transmission. Infected breeder birds may harbor the pathogen in reproductive organs, leading to contamination of eggs during formation and subsequent infection of chicks upon hatching. This vertical transmission contributes to persistent flock-level infection. Horizontal transmission within grow-out houses further amplifies the spread. Studies have shown that *Salmonella* serovars isolated from processing plant carcasses often match those from breeder flocks, indicating a direct link [35, 36]. Thus, breeder flocks play a critical role in the sustained presence of *Salmonella* in broiler production. In vertically integrated broiler systems, hatcheries can serve as significant reservoirs for *Salmonella*, with contamination often traced to this early stage. Infected hatcheries can transmit the pathogen through eggs, leading to colonization in newly hatched chicks [37, 38]. *Salmonella* can persist as an endemic population within hatchery environments, continually infecting new flocks. Day-old chicks are particularly vulnerable due to their immature gut microbiota and low resistance to infection, making early colonization a critical concern for downstream contamination [39].

Eggs may become contaminated with *Salmonella*—most commonly *S.* Enteritidis—by two principal pathways: vertical (trans-ovarial) and horizontal (fecal-oral). When the hen's ovary or oviduct is colonized by *S.* Enteritidis, bacteria can be deposited directly into the developing yolk, vitelline membrane, or albumen before the shell forms. Thus, the organism is already inside the egg during the time of lay [40]. In contrast, fecal-oral spread originates in the intestinal tract. During or after oviposition, *Salmonella* present in feces or contaminated litter can penetrate the porous, incompletely cured cuticle of a freshly laid egg. Shell invasion is most efficient within the first minutes post-lay, when cuticular maturation is incomplete and pore channels remain open [41]. Environmental contamination of nest boxes and hatcheries further facilitates outer-shell seeding. Although shell thickness per se is not consistently linked to the likelihood of penetration by *S.* Typhimurium, eggs with higher specific-gravity shells exhibit greater resistance to invasion by *S.* Enteritidis [40].

5.2 Insects

Insect and vertebrate vectors constitute major routes for *Salmonella* introduction into feed, poultry flocks, and, ultimately, humans. Cockroaches can carry foodborne pathogens such as *Salmonella* into poultry houses, where their movements and contact with flock mates enable cross-contamination and subsequent spread of the bacteria among previously uninfected birds [42]. Experiments conducted by Leffer et al. showed that *S.* Enteritidis-infected *Alphitobius diaperinus* (both adult insects and larvae) were capable of transmitting the bacteria into the chicks. The study also showed that the concentration of *Salmonella* Enteritidis recovered from the cecum, liver, or spleen of experimental chicks was larger in birds that had been fed infected larvae than in those that had received infected adult insects [43]. Flies recovered from poultry houses frequently carry *Salmonella*, and the poultry red mite *Dermanyssus gallinae* has likewise been identified as a biological vector for *S.* Enteritidis within these facilities. Chicks may become infected either by ingesting crushed, contaminated mites or through exposure to mites during their blood-feeding activity, both of which introduce the pathogen into the flock [44].

5.3 Feed

Salmonella is frequently detected in various feed ingredients—both animal- and plant-derived proteins such as soybean meal, rapeseed, palm kernel, rice bran, and cottonseed. Consequently, compound feed represents a major pathway for introducing novel *Salmonella* infections into livestock populations, especially poultry. In numerous instances, the same serovars isolated from raw feed components have been traced through processing to the finished feed. Case-control investigations have also linked particular ingredients to salmonellosis outbreaks, although detection of *Salmonella* in feed does not always coincide with clinical disease [45].

5.4 Trade and travel

On-farm pathogen-control programs aim to deliver birds to the plant free of detectable *Salmonella*. Yet the stresses of feed withdrawal, catching, and transport—combined with dirty crates, trucks, and crews—can spread enteric bacteria through contamination and cross-contamination. To curb *Salmonella* before slaughter, it is vital to minimize birds' exposure in the final hours during loading, transit, and holding. Studying how quickly *Salmonella* moves from the environment to birds in this window could reveal a key control point for cutting the number of infected chickens that reach the plant [46].

6. *Salmonella* behavior in different poultry matrices

6.1 Fresh meat vs. processed products

Fresh poultry meat presents a highly perishable environment with a near-neutral pH (~6.0), high water activity (aw > 0.98), and abundant nutrients—ideal conditions for *Salmonella* survival and growth. A considerably higher rate of *Salmonella* contamination in fresh chicken meat sold in wet markets could result from relatively poor hygiene practices, such as sharing a knife and cutting board without properly cleaning them and putting chicken carcasses in the chillers without physical separation or individual packaging [47]. The potential for *Salmonella* spp. to contaminate household environments has been well documented. Gorman et al. highlighted that the handling and preparation of raw foods, particularly fresh poultry such as chicken, significantly increases the risk of *Salmonella* dissemination to hands and food-contact surfaces [48]. Cross-contamination within domestic kitchens accounts for a considerable proportion of foodborne transmission events. Multiple studies have demonstrated that *Salmonella* cells originating from frozen broiler chickens are capable of contaminating food preparation environments [49]. De Boer and Hahne [50] further confirmed the ease with which *Salmonella* can be transferred from raw poultry to various kitchen surfaces, utensils, hands, and subsequently to other foods. Notably, viable *Salmonella* cells have been recovered from contaminated surfaces for up to 6 hours post-exposure, underscoring the pathogen's persistence in the domestic environment [50]. Post-slaughter interventions like chilling reduce microbial load but do not eliminate the pathogen.

A very small proportion of the overall consumption now consists of whole chicken as compared to the 1980s (almost 50%). For instance, in 2015, chickens sold in the United States as whole carcasses, cut pieces, or processed products accounted for 11%, 40%, and 49% of total sales, respectively. Poultry processed products fall into four major categories—Breaded (cordon bleus, wiener schnitzel, and nuggets), deli meats (ham, pâtés, terrines, rillettes, sausages, and galantine), cured, marinated, or raw (cut-up pieces, skewers, chopped, and stuffed products), and cooked (preserved and roasted meat) [51]. Various human cases of *Salmonella* Enteritidis infections linked to uncooked, frozen, breaded chicken items were documented in Canada by Hobbs et al. [52] and Morton et al. [53]. Different strains of *Salmonella* (Heidelberg, Enteritidis, and Orion) were found in raw frozen chicken nuggets and strips in Canada by Bucher et al. [54]. Eglezos et al. examined the bacteriological quality of 300 batches of raw, frozen chicken nuggets produced over a 4-year period in Queensland, Australia and the prevalence of *Salmonella* spp. was estimated to be 8.7% of the population [55].

6.2 Marinated, frozen, and vacuum-packed poultry

Marination, commonly performed with acidic solutions containing vinegar, citric acid, or phosphates, can influence *Salmonella* survival. Marination processes utilizing natural ingredients rich in organic acids or essential oils (EOs) have been shown to effectively inhibit the growth of common foodborne pathogens, including *Campylobacter* spp. and *Salmonella* spp., in poultry meat, and may also facilitate their inactivation [56]. The combination of a cultured sugar and vinegar blend with commercial seasoning shows potential as an effective strategy for controlling *Salmonella* Typhimurium in poultry products during refrigerated storage. Furthermore, the application of a 3% cultured sugar and vinegar blend mitigated texture degradation in frozen chicken breasts and enhanced the tenderness of refrigerated, ready-to-eat chicken breasts—an attribute frequently regarded as the most critical quality parameter for both refrigerated and frozen poultry products [57]. *Salmonella* contamination in frozen poultry products remains a significant public health concern. Despite freezing, *Salmonella* can survive in frozen poultry, posing a risk if the product is improperly cooked. Studies have shown that *Salmonella* can persist during frozen storage, with some cells becoming structurally injured but still viable [58]. Prevalence studies indicate that *Salmonella* can be found in frozen poultry products. For instance, a study in England found *Salmonella* in 8.8% of frozen, reformed chicken products. Another study reported a 7.6% prevalence in frozen chicken parts [59, 60]. Vacuum packaging creates an anaerobic environment, which does not inherently inhibit *Salmonella*, as many strains are facultative anaerobes. However, the reduced oxygen availability can limit spoilage organisms, indirectly affecting microbial competition. Modified atmosphere packaging (MAP), incorporating CO_2 or N_2, may further influence microbial dynamics, though studies show variable efficacy depending on gas ratios and storage temperature [61].

6.3 Egg-based matrices

Eggs and egg-based products continue to be a major vehicle for *Salmonella* transmission, particularly in the European Union (EU), where in 2018, 45.6% of reported salmonellosis outbreaks were attributed to their consumption [62, 63]. *Salmonella* Enteritidis is the predominant serovar implicated in egg-associated human infections [64]. Contamination levels within intact eggs are generally low, typically below 10 CFU/egg [65, 66]; however, significantly higher counts (e.g., >10^5 CFU/g) have also been detected [66]. The albumen is more frequently contaminated than the yolk, indicating colonization of the oviduct during egg formation [67]. Despite the presence of *Salmonella*, growth within albumen is typically inhibited due to its inherent antimicrobial properties, even at ambient temperatures [68, 69]. In contrast, the yolk can support rapid bacterial proliferation, with generation times as short as 35 minutes at 37°C. Growth has been observed at 10°C in some studies, although not consistently. Storage temperatures of 8°C or lower appear to suppress *Salmonella* growth effectively [70].

Surveillance data indicate that the prevalence of *Salmonella* in commercially produced table eggs is relatively low in developed countries. In the United States, the estimated contamination rate is approximately 0.005% [71], while in Europe, the European Food Safety Authority (EFSA) and ECDC reported a prevalence of 0.37% based on testing of over 6000 eggs [63]. However, a higher risk has been observed with home-produced or backyard eggs. Several outbreaks have been associated with backyard poultry and the consumption of home-laid eggs [72, 73]. In one study, 10.4% of samples from backyard flocks tested positive for *Salmonella* [74]. Additional risk factors include the use of pooled raw eggs in dishes like dressings, desserts, and custards, some of which may not undergo sufficient thermal processing [75–77]. Common contributing factors to outbreaks include undercooking, inadequate storage, and cross-contamination [78, 79]. Outbreaks have occurred in both private and public settings, often involving contaminated eggs or raw-egg-based dishes [80].

7. Biofilm formation in poultry-associated environments

A biofilm comprises microorganisms that adhere irreversibly to biotic or abiotic interfaces—and to one another—while being enveloped in their own extracellular polymeric matrix [81]. *Salmonella* spp. form biofilms both within hosts and in external habitats; however, this phenotype is particularly critical for persistence under non-host conditions. Biofilm formation underpins the organism's widespread environmental distribution, facilitating its recovery from water, soil, and plant surfaces. Extensive experimental evidence shows that *Salmonella* readily colonizes and establishes biofilms on a range of abiotic substrates commonly encountered on farms, in abattoirs, and throughout food-processing facilities, including plastic, rubber, glass, stainless steel, and cement [82]. Within the poultry production chain, *Salmonella* biofilms constitute a major reservoir of contamination. Accumulating evidence demonstrates that such biofilms underlie persistent *Salmonella* colonization of hatchery incubators, farm water-distribution systems, and live-bird transport vehicles [83, 84].

8. Detection and quantification of *Salmonella* in poultry matrices

8.1 Traditional culture methods

Traditional methods remain the gold standard for detecting *Salmonella* due to their high specificity and ability to confirm viable organisms. Conventional methods for bacterial isolation rely on culturing samples on differential agar media followed by colony enumeration. The standard protocol for detecting *Salmonella* in food involves several key steps: pre-enrichment in buffered peptone water, selective enrichment, isolation on differential media, and serological confirmation, as outlined in the NF EN ISO 6579 standard. While widely used, these procedures are labor-intensive, time-consuming, and often challenging to interpret. Initial results typically require 2–4 days, with an additional 4–6 days needed for confirmatory testing. During this period, the affected food products cannot be released for commercial distribution [85].

8.2 Molecular and rapid detection techniques

The application of advanced molecular techniques in the characterization of microbial populations associated with poultry meat has significantly enhanced our understanding of microbial ecology and pathogen behavior during various stages of poultry processing. Traditional culture-based methods, while valuable, are often limited in their ability to detect the full spectrum of microbial diversity, particularly in complex environments such as poultry processing facilities. In contrast, molecular tools such as denaturing gradient gel electrophoresis (DGGE), multiplex polymerase chain reaction (PCR), quantitative PCR (qPCR), and next-generation sequencing (NGS) have enabled high-resolution analysis of microbial communities, including non-culturable and low-abundance species.

These methods are especially useful for monitoring changes in microbial communities and progression patterns in response to processing interventions (such as chilling, scalding, and antimicrobial treatments), equipment sanitation, and environmental conditions. For example, DGGE can provide rapid fingerprinting of community profiles, while qPCR offers quantification of specific pathogens or functional genes. NGS, with its ability to generate comprehensive taxonomic and functional profiles, has emerged as a powerful tool for microbiome studies in poultry meat and processing environments. This includes identification of core microbiota, detection of spoilage organisms, and surveillance of antimicrobial resistance genes.

As NGS becomes increasingly cost-effective and user-friendly, its application in poultry microbiome research is expanding rapidly. Microbiome mapping of poultry carcasses, processing equipment surfaces, water systems, and air samples within facilities allows for the generation of detailed datasets that capture spatial and temporal microbial dynamics. These analyses can reveal previously unrecognized sources of cross-contamination, identify persistent microbial reservoirs within the plant, and elucidate the influence of external factors such as geographic location, farm management practices, and flock health on the microbial landscape of processing environments.

Furthermore, understanding these microbial patterns has practical implications for food safety and quality. Microbial community profiles can be linked to spoilage potential and shelf-life outcomes, informing risk-based decision-making. Importantly, this level of microbial resolution supports the development of targeted, facility-specific sanitation and intervention strategies. By tailoring control measures to the unique microbial signature of each processing plant, processors may achieve greater efficacy in reducing contamination, improving product quality, and enhancing overall food safety outcomes [86].

9. Epidemiology of *Salmonella* outbreaks linked to poultry

Salmonella continues to be a leading cause of foodborne illness worldwide, with poultry products frequently implicated. Between 1990 and 2014, a total of 53 outbreaks of live poultry-associated salmonellosis (LPAS) were reported in the United States, resulting in 2630 documented illnesses, 387 hospitalizations, and 5 fatalities. The median age of affected individuals was 9 years, with a reported age range from less than 1 year to 92 years. Exposure to chicks and ducklings was identified in 85% and 38% of cases, respectively. Notably, certain high-risk behaviors were frequently observed, including housing live poultry indoors (46% of cases) and kissing birds (13%) [87]. In 2021, an outbreak of *Salmonella* Hader associated with ground turkey was reported, resulting in 33 confirmed cases and 4 hospitalizations [88]. That same year, an outbreak of *Salmonella* Enteritidis was linked to raw frozen breaded stuffed chicken products, with 36 reported infections and 12 hospitalizations across 11 states [89]. Additionally, one of the recent outbreaks associated with backyard poultry occurred in 2021, leading to 1135 cases, 273 hospitalizations, and 2 fatalities. The Center for Disease Control and Prevention (CDC) reported that 25% of the affected individuals were children under the age of five [90]. Trends show seasonal peaks in warmer months and rising incidence in low- and middle-income countries due to limited regulation.

9.1 Serotype distribution in poultry-linked outbreaks

The most frequently isolated *Salmonella* serotypes from chicken include *S.* Kentucky, *S.* Enteritidis, *S.* Typhimurium, *S.* Infantis, and *S.* Heidelberg. In turkeys, the predominant serotypes identified were *S.* Reading, *S.* Kentucky, *S.* Agona, *S.* Hadar, and *S.* Ouakam. Among human cases of salmonellosis, the most commonly implicated serotypes are *S.* Enteritidis, *S.* Typhimurium, *S.* Newport, *S.* I4,[5],12:i:-, *S.* Javiana, and *S.* Heidelberg. Notably, *S.* Heidelberg has demonstrated elevated resistance to two or more antibiotics, regardless of whether the source was from conventionally or organically raised poultry [91]. Multidrug-resistant (MDR) *Salmonella* was more prevalent in isolates obtained from retail ground turkey (36%) compared to those from retail chicken (20%). Additionally, antimicrobial-resistant (AMR) *Salmonella* isolates from turkeys demonstrated a higher rate of resistance to three or more antimicrobial classes (46.7%) than isolates from chickens (14.6%) collected *via* the cecal sampling route [92]. *Salmonella* Heidelberg isolates linked to the 2011 ground turkey outbreak were found to harbor a novel virulence plasmid encoding the VirB4/D4 type IV secretion system. This secretion system enhances the pathogen's ability to invade and persist within macrophages and intestinal epithelial cells, thereby contributing to increased virulence [93, 94]. In 2011, a significant outbreak of *Salmonella* Heidelberg was reported, resulting in 190 confirmed cases and 30 hospitalizations. The outbreak was traced back to Kosher broiled chicken livers, highlighting the potential risks associated with partially cooked poultry products. During the same year, multistate outbreaks of *Salmonella* Altona and *Salmonella* Johannesburg occurred in the United States, leading to 68 infections and 19 hospitalizations. Epidemiological investigations linked these infections to contact with live poultry, specifically chicks and ducklings [95]. Additionally, an outbreak of *Salmonella* Hadar was documented in 2011, affecting 12 individuals, three of whom required hospitalization. The *S.* Hadar strain involved in this outbreak exhibited multidrug resistance, including resistance to ampicillin, amoxicillin/clavulanate, cephalothin, and tetracycline, raising concerns about treatment challenges and antimicrobial resistance in zoonotic pathogens [96].

10. Intervention strategies in the poultry chain

Effective control of *Salmonella* in poultry production requires a multi-hurdle approach encompassing all stages of the supply chain. On-farm interventions are crucial for reducing the initial bacterial load before birds reach processing facilities. Vaccination, particularly against *Salmonella* Enteritidis, has been instrumental in lowering contamination in breeder and layer flocks. The implementation of live and inactivated vaccines has led to substantial reductions in vertical transmission [97, 98]. In addition, the use of competitive exclusion cultures and probiotics promotes gut microbiota stability, thereby inhibiting *Salmonella* colonization through microbial antagonism and immune modulation [99]. Biosecurity measures, including restricted farm access, controlled feed and water sources, and stringent sanitation protocols, are also vital in preventing environmental and cross-flock contamination [100].

Within processing plants, various interventions are applied to further reduce microbial loads. Thermal treatments such as scalding, as well as carcass rinses using chlorinated water or organic acid solutions, are commonly employed to inactivate *Salmonella*. Among chemical decontaminants, peracetic acid has gained widespread use due to its efficacy and minimal residual impact [101]. Separating zones of hygiene, staff training, and strict segregation of raw and cooked products are essential for preventing cross-contamination within facilities [102]. These process control strategies are often monitored under Hazard Analysis and Critical Control Points (HACCP) systems to ensure regulatory compliance and food safety assurance [103].

Post-processing interventions are increasingly focused on minimizing recontamination and enhancing product shelf-life. Packaging technologies such as modified atmosphere packaging (MAP), which alters the gaseous environment surrounding the product, can significantly reduce microbial growth [104]. Antimicrobial packaging films embedded with agents like nisin or organic acids further inhibit bacterial proliferation [105]. For ready-to-eat (RTE) poultry products, high-pressure processing (HPP) and irradiation are being explored for their ability to inactivate pathogens without compromising sensory quality [106]. These innovations hold promise in extending safety measures beyond the processing plant and into the retail and consumer environment.

Ultimately, the integration of on-farm controls, processing plant interventions, and post-processing technologies forms a comprehensive framework to mitigate *Salmonella* risk in poultry products. Continuous evaluation and adaptation of these strategies, in response to evolving pathogen profiles and consumer demands, remain essential for maintaining food safety across the poultry supply chain.

11. Regulatory frameworks and industry standards

The Healthy People 2030 initiative aims to reduce the national incidence of *Salmonella* infections by 25%. Given that poultry—particularly chicken and turkey—is a significant source of human salmonellosis, the US Department of Agriculture (USDA) Food Safety and Inspection Service (FSIS) has proposed a new *Salmonella* Control Framework targeting a 25% reduction in poultry-attributable salmonellosis cases. A key component of this framework is a Final Product Standard, which deems raw chicken carcasses, chicken parts, comminuted chicken, and comminuted turkey to be adulterated if they meet both of the following criteria:

1. Contain *Salmonella* at or above 10 CFU/mL or 10 CFU/g, and

2. Contain any detectable level of at least one *Salmonella* serotype of public health concern specific to that product type.

Additionally, the framework proposes implementing a Statistical Process Control (SPC) program aimed at improving processing hygiene. This includes achieving at least a 1-log reduction in aerobic plate counts (AC) between two designated sampling points within the processing plant [107].

National and international *Salmonella* control programs have been established to address the significant public health risks associated with *Salmonella* contamination in poultry. These programs, coordinated by government agencies and international organizations such as the World Health Organization (WHO), the Codex Alimentarius Commission, and the World Organization for Animal Health (WOAH), implement harmonized strategies aimed at reducing *Salmonella* prevalence throughout the poultry production chain [108]. In the European Union (EU), a comprehensive control framework mandates routine testing for high-risk serovars like *Salmonella* Enteritidis and *S.* Typhimurium, vaccination of laying hens, and strict biosecurity practices across member states [109]. Similarly, in the United States, the National Poultry Improvement Plan (NPIP) offers a widely adopted voluntary certification system, while the Food and Drug Administration (FDA) enforces the mandatory egg safety rule for commercial layer flocks to detect and manage *S.* Enteritidis contamination. Core components of these programs include routine surveillance and monitoring, which allow for early detection and corrective action, as well as robust data collection to inform national food safety strategies. Vaccination is another critical preventive measure, particularly for breeder and layer flocks, although policies vary by country based on vaccine efficacy in field conditions. Biosecurity remains a foundational element, with protocols in place to prevent horizontal and vertical transmission *via* sanitation, pest control, and movement restrictions. Certification and quality assurance mechanisms help validate compliance, improving market access and consumer confidence. Additionally, national and regional surveillance systems such as the European Food Safety Authority (EFSA) database and the U.S. CDC's PulseNet and FoodNet networks monitor disease trends and detect outbreaks. Investment in research and development continues to enhance control measures through new vaccine technologies, biosecurity innovations, and alternatives to antibiotics, addressing antimicrobial resistance (AMR) concerns. Educational outreach to farmers further supports these efforts by promoting best practices and enhancing program adoption. Some countries also encourage the use of alternative pathogen-control methods, including probiotics, organic acids, and other microbiome-supportive approaches, to reduce reliance on antibiotics. Collectively, these integrated programs play a pivotal role in mitigating the burden of *Salmonella* infections, promoting food safety, and supporting the sustainable production and global trade of poultry products [110].

12. Consumer awareness and education

Consumer awareness and education are vital components of a comprehensive strategy to reduce the risk of *Salmonella* infections originating from poultry products. As poultry is frequently implicated in foodborne disease outbreaks, the role of the end-user—primarily households—becomes a critical control point in the farm-to-fork continuum. Despite extensive regulatory and industry interventions aimed at reducing contamination at the production and processing levels, improper food handling at the consumer level remains a significant contributor to disease burden [111].

One of the fundamental areas of focus is the promotion of safe handling and cooking practices. Public health agencies such as the Center for Disease Control and Prevention (CDC), US Department of Agriculture (USDA), and international counterparts emphasize the need to cook poultry products to an internal temperature of at least 74°C (165°F) to ensure microbial safety [112]. Additionally, consumers are advised to store raw poultry at or below 4°C (40°F), avoid washing raw meat (which can spread pathogens through aerosolized droplets), and prevent cross-contamination by using separate utensils and cutting boards for raw and ready-to-eat foods [113]. Despite the clarity and consistency of these messages, behavioral adherence remains inconsistent. Research has demonstrated that only a minority of consumers regularly use food thermometers to verify doneness, instead relying on subjective indicators such as color or texture, which can be misleading [114]. This discrepancy underscores a persistent gap between food safety knowledge and actual kitchen practices.

To address these issues, clear labeling and public health campaigns have been implemented to enhance consumer understanding and engagement [115]. Accurate and visible labeling—such as "raw," "partially cooked," or "ready-to-eat" (RTE)—on poultry packaging is essential to inform consumer decision-making. Misinterpretation of labeling can result in undercooking or mishandling of products, especially with items that appear cooked (e.g., breaded or grilled poultry products) (https://www.fsis.usda.gov/guidelines/2017-0017). Public awareness campaigns like "Fight BAC!" by the Partnership for Food Safety Education have played a crucial role in promoting hygienic practices through the "Clean, Separate, Cook, and Chill" framework [116]. These campaigns aim to simplify complex microbiological concepts into actionable behaviors and have reached broad audiences through schools, healthcare settings, media, and community events.

Beyond traditional education, recent efforts have turned to behavioral science-based interventions to more effectively modify consumer habits. Behavioral economics and cognitive psychology suggest that information alone is often insufficient to drive change; instead, structural nudges and environmental cues can more effectively prompt safer behaviors. For example, point-of-sale prompts, instructional graphics on product packaging, and short instructional videos placed near refrigerated poultry displays have all been evaluated for their impact on consumer compliance with food safety guidelines. Some interventions leverage "default settings" or simplify decision-making, such as including integrated color-change indicators or embedded thermometers in packaging. These tactics aim to reduce the cognitive and practical barriers consumers face in applying food safety practices [117].

Despite ongoing efforts, several barriers still limit the effectiveness of consumer food safety education. Cultural norms, language differences, and low levels of food literacy can make it difficult for messages to reach and influence all audiences. Additionally, people's perception of risk often differs across demographic groups, which affects their motivation to follow safe food handling practices. To improve outcomes, food safety messages should be tailored to account for social and cultural diversity and specifically target high-risk groups, such as households with young children, elderly individuals, or those with weakened immune systems.

13. Control strategies for *Salmonella* in poultry

Implementing strong biosecurity measures—such as site cleanliness, hand hygiene, disinfection between flocks, and pest control—is essential for reducing *Salmonella* transmission in poultry farms. Proper litter management, including composting, and the use of effective disinfectants also help lower contamination. Seasonal variations, with higher prevalence in summer, further emphasize the need for year-round biosecurity vigilance [118, 119]. Prebiotics such as Yeast cell wall-derived mannan oligosaccharides (MOS), fructo-oligosaccharides (FOS), inulin, and xylo-oligosaccharides help control *Salmonella* in poultry by promoting SCFA production (e.g., butyrate and acetate) in the ceca, which lowers gut pH and inhibits pathogen colonization [120] Probiotics, or direct-fed microbials (DFM), are live microorganisms that, when given in adequate amounts, provide health benefits to the host, as defined by the FAO [121]. Continuous supplementation with Bacillus-based probiotics has been shown to restore gut microbiota, reduce *Salmonella* load in internal organs, and increase butyrate levels in free-laying birds challenged with *S.* Typhimurium [122]. Bacteriophage therapy has shown promise in reducing *Salmonella* colonization and improving survival in infected poultry. Phage cocktails (e.g., F1055S and F12013S) sprayed on eggs reduced horizontal transmission [123], while oral or injected phages lowered bacterial loads in internal organs and alleviated clinical symptoms [124]. Broad-host-range phages offer added benefits by targeting multiple *Salmonella* serovars. Encapsulation techniques help protect phages from degradation in the acidic gastric environment, enhancing their oral efficacy [125].

Live attenuated vaccines contain living bacterial pathogens that have been weakened or rendered non-virulent through attenuation techniques, including chemical treatment or genetic modification [126]. Shin et al. evaluated the immune response and protective efficacy of a temperature-sensitive attenuated *Salmonella* Enteritidis mutant as a potential live vaccine candidate. Additionally, they also investigated the impact of different vaccination strategies to enhance both humoral and cellular immunity in chickens. Two administration regimens were compared: the oral/IM group received an oral dose at 4 weeks of age followed by an intramuscular booster at 7 weeks, while the IM/oral group received the reverse sequence. The oral/IM group demonstrated stronger immune responses than the IM/oral group. Furthermore, spleen samples from the oral/IM group showed a notable reduction in *Salmonella* load following challenge. These findings support the potential of the attenuated *S.* Enteritidis mutant as an effective live vaccine candidate [127]. The study by Lin et al. assessed the safety and efficacy of the commercial bivalent live attenuated vaccine *AviPro Salmonella DUO* in both SPF (specific pathogen free) chickens and commercial layer hens. The vaccine was found to be safe, with no adverse effects on bird health, and showed protective effects against *Salmonella* Enteritidis (SE) and *S.* Typhimurium (ST). Vaccinated layers had lower mortality and higher egg production compared to unvaccinated controls. *Salmonella* shedding and tissue colonization were significantly reduced after a single dose, while triple vaccination fully inhibited cloacal shedding and markedly decreased bacterial loads in tissues. These findings support the vaccine's potential as an effective component of integrated *Salmonella* control strategies in poultry production [97].

Killed (inactivated) bacterin vaccines, produced using whole-cell *Salmonella* preparations treated with agents such as heat, formaldehyde, or radiation, have been widely applied to control *Salmonella* infections in poultry. These vaccines primarily induce humoral immunity and typically require booster doses due to limited cell-mediated immune response. Despite this limitation, they are favored over live vaccines in certain settings due to improved biosecurity and safety profiles [128]. Multivalent formulations are often necessary to target diverse circulating serovars. Notably, a trivalent aluminum hydroxide-adjuvanted vaccine significantly reduced *Salmonella* Enteritidis and *S.* Infantis loads and prevented liver dissemination. Enhanced antibody responses and broader protection were observed when live and killed vaccines were used in combination [129].

Efforts to develop subunit vaccines against *Salmonella* Enteritidis in poultry have focused on components such as outer membrane proteins (OMPs), flagellins, fimbrial proteins, and secretory system effectors. OMPs like OmpC and OmpF have demonstrated strong immunogenicity and, when administered using a booster strategy, conferred high levels of protection in young chickens [130]. Flagellar protein FliC elicited robust antibody responses but failed to induce cellular immunity, offering limited protection [131]. More recently, outer membrane vesicles (OMVs), which carry surface antigens and can stimulate both humoral and cellular responses, have emerged as promising subunit vaccine candidates [132]. OMVs alone provided 90% protection, and when combined with purified OmpF, achieved complete protection against *S.* Enteritidis in vaccinated birds [130].

14. Gaps in knowledge and future research directions

Despite considerable advances in the control and understanding of *Salmonella* in poultry production, critical knowledge gaps persist that hinder the development of more effective risk mitigation strategies. One major limitation lies in the reliance on generalized risk models that fail to account for the diverse nature of poultry products. Current assessments often treat poultry matrices homogenously, overlooking the unique characteristics of products such as mechanically separated meat, marinated cuts, or ready-to-eat poultry items. These matrix-specific factors—such as pH, water activity, and marinade composition—can significantly influence *Salmonella* behavior, survival, and growth. To enhance risk characterization and predictive modeling, future research must prioritize the development of matrix-specific quantitative microbial risk assessment (QMRA) models tailored to individual poultry product types [133].

Another underexplored area is the role of sub-lethal injury and stress adaptation in *Salmonella* survival. During processing and storage, *Salmonella* cells may undergo sub-lethal stress (e.g., due to heat, cold, desiccation, or sanitizers), leading to a physiological state that hampers detection by conventional microbiological methods. However, these injured cells may regain viability under favorable conditions, posing a latent risk to public health. Understanding the molecular mechanisms underlying stress responses, persistence, and recovery in different poultry matrices is essential to improving detection methods and refining hazard assessments [134].

Finally, addressing *Salmonella* risks requires a holistic One Health approach that integrates human, animal, and environmental health domains. The complex

DOI: http://dx.doi.org/10.5772/intechopen.1012025

transmission routes of *Salmonella*—from farm environments and animal reservoirs to processing plants and consumers—necessitate interdisciplinary collaboration. Moreover, the growing concern over antimicrobial resistance (AMR) in *Salmonella* further highlights the need for surveillance systems and control strategies that consider the interconnectedness of the ecosystem. Coordinated efforts across sectors are crucial to reducing the burden of *Salmonella* infections and curbing the emergence and dissemination of resistant strains [135].

15. Conclusion

The role of poultry matrices in the transmission of *Salmonella* encompasses complex interactions between microbial physiology, food matrix characteristics, and environmental conditions encountered along the production and distribution continuum. The survival, persistence, and potential proliferation of *Salmonella* within specific matrices—such as raw carcass parts, mechanically separated meat, marinated or frozen products, and ready-to-eat formulations—are governed by a combination of intrinsic (e.g., pH, water activity, and nutrient availability) and extrinsic (e.g., temperature, packaging atmosphere, and storage duration) factors. Despite advances in pre-harvest and post-harvest control strategies—including vaccination, decontamination technologies, and regulatory oversight—matrix-specific risks remain insufficiently characterized. Current risk assessment models often fail to account for the heterogeneity of poultry matrices, potentially underestimating the public health risk posed by certain processed or value-added products. Furthermore, the emergence of antimicrobial-resistant and highly adapted *Salmonella* serotypes underscores the need for continuous surveillance and refinement of intervention approaches.

To enhance food safety outcomes, future research should prioritize the development of matrix-specific quantitative microbial risk assessment (QMRA) frameworks, improved detection methodologies capable of identifying sub-lethally injured or viable but non-culturable (VBNC) *Salmonella* cells, and a deeper understanding of the molecular mechanisms governing matrix-pathogen interactions. Integrated, systems-based approaches that consider the entire supply chain—from primary production through to consumer behavior—are essential for the development of targeted, evidence-based mitigation strategies. Through a more nuanced understanding of poultry matrices as ecological niches for *Salmonella*, it is possible to more effectively reduce the burden of foodborne salmonellosis.

Author details

Greeshma Bharathan and Shabarinath Srikumar*
Department of Poultry Science, College of Agriculture, Auburn University, Alabama, USA

*Address all correspondence to: szs0397@auburn.edu

References

[1] Grimont PA, Weill F-X. Antigenic Formulae of the *Salmonella* Serovars. 9th ed. WHO Collaborating Centre for Reference Research on Salmonella; 2007. pp. 1-166

[2] Havelaar AH, Kirk MD, Torgerson PR, Gibb HJ, Hald T, Lake RJ, et al. World Health Organization global estimates and regional comparisons of the burden of foodborne disease in 2010. PLoS Medicine. 2015;**12**(12):e1001923

[3] European Food Safety Authority, European Centre for Disease Prevention and Control. The European Union summary report on trends and sources of zoonoses, zoonotic agents and food-borne outbreaks in 2017. EFSA Journal. 2018;**16**(12):e05500

[4] Mumy KL. *Salmonella*. In: Wexler P, editor. Encyclopedia of Toxicology. 3rd ed. Oxford: Academic Press; 2014. pp. 211-212

[5] Mølbak K, Olsen JE, Wegener HC. *Salmonella* infections. In: Foodborne Infections and Intoxications. Elsevier; 2006. pp. 57-136

[6] Uzzau S, Brown DJ, Wallis T, Rubino S, Leori G, Bernard S, et al. Host adapted serotypes of *Salmonella enterica*. Epidemiology and Infection. 2000;**125**(2):229-255

[7] Tamber S. *Salmonella*. In: Dikeman M, editor. Encyclopedia of Meat Sciences. 3rd ed. Oxford: Elsevier; 2024. pp. 275-287

[8] Foster JW, Hall HK. Inducible pH homeostasis and the acid tolerance response of *Salmonella* Typhimurium. Journal of Bacteriology. 1991;**173**(16):5129-5135

[9] Fàbrega A, Vila J. *Salmonella enterica* serovar Typhimurium skills to succeed in the host: Virulence and regulation. Clinical Microbiology Reviews. 2013;**26**(2):308-341

[10] Takeuchi A. Electron microscope studies of experimental *Salmonella* infection. I. Penetration into the intestinal epithelium by *Salmonella* Typhimurium. The American Journal of Pathology. 1967;**50**(1):109

[11] Sansonetti P. Host–pathogen interactions: The seduction of molecular cross talk. Gut. 2002;**50**(suppl 3):iii2-iii8

[12] Wagner C, Hensel M. Adhesive mechanisms of *Salmonella enterica*. In: Bacterial Adhesion: Chemistry, Biology and Physics. Springer; 2011. pp. 17-34

[13] Hafez MM, Aboulwafa MM, Yassien MA, Hassouna NA. Role of different classes of mammalian cell surface molecules in adherence of coagulase positive and coagulase negative *Staphylococci*. Journal of Basic Microbiology. 2008;**48**(5):353-362

[14] Henry-Stanley MJ, Hess DJ, Erlandsen SL, Wells CL. Ability of the heparan sulfate proteoglycan syndecan-1 to participate in bacterial translocation across the intestinal epithelial barrier. Shock. 2005;**24**(6):571-576

[15] Rajas O, Quirós LM, Ortega M, Vazquez-Espinosa E, Merayo-Lloves J, Vazquez F, et al. Glycosaminoglycans are involved in bacterial adherence to lung cells. BMC Infectious Diseases. 2017;**17**(1):1-14

[16] Rehman T, Yin L, Latif MB, Chen J, Wang K, Geng Y, et al. Adhesive mechanism of different

Salmonella fimbrial adhesins. Microbial Pathogenesis. 2019;**137**:103748

[17] Francis C, Starnbach M, Falkow S. Morphological and cytoskeletal changes in epithelial cells occur immediately upon interaction with *Salmonella* Typhimurium grown under low-oxygen conditions. Molecular Microbiology. 1992;**6**(21):3077-3087

[18] Merino L, Procura F, Trejo FM, Bueno DJ, Golowczyc MA. Biofilm formation by *Salmonella* sp. in the poultry industry: Detection, control and eradication strategies. Food Research International. 2019;**119**:530-540

[19] Humphries AD, Raffatellu M, Winter S, Weening EH, Kingsley RA, Droleskey R, et al. The use of flow cytometry to detect expression of subunits encoded by 11 *Salmonella enterica* serotype Typhimurium fimbrial operons. Molecular Microbiology. 2003;**48**(5):1357-1376

[20] Collinson S, Doig P, Doran J, Clouthier S, Trust T, Kay W. Thin, aggregative fimbriae mediate binding of *Salmonella* enteritidis to fibronectin. Journal of Bacteriology. 1993;**175**(1):12-18

[21] Galán JE. *Salmonella* Typhimurium and inflammation: A pathogen-centric affair. Nature Reviews Microbiology. 2021;**19**(11):716-725

[22] Rogers AW, Tsolis RM, Bäumler AJ. *Salmonella* versus the microbiome. Microbiology and Molecular Biology Reviews. 17 Feb 2021;**85**(1):10-128

[23] Wotzka SY, Nguyen BD, Hardt W-D. *Salmonella* Typhimurium diarrhea reveals basic principles of enteropathogen infection and disease-promoted DNA exchange. Cell Host & Microbe. 2017;**21**(4):443-454

[24] Rajashekar R, Liebl D, Seitz A, Hensel M. Dynamic remodeling of the endosomal system during formation of *Salmonella*-induced filaments by intracellular *Salmonella enterica*. Traffic. 2008;**9**(12):2100-2116

[25] Kumar P, Verma AK, Umaraw P, Mehta N, Sazili AQ. Processing and preparation of slaughtered poultry. In: Postharvest and Postmortem Processing of Raw Food Materials. Woodhead Publishing, Elsevier; 2022. pp. 281-314

[26] Featherstone S. 2 - Food regulations, standards, and labelling. In: Featherstone S, editor. A Complete Course in Canning and Related Processes. 14th ed. Cambridge, UK: Woodhead Publishing; 2015. pp. 21-61

[27] Cavani C, Petracci M, Trocino A, Xiccato G. Advances in research on poultry and rabbit meat quality. Italian Journal of Animal Science. 2009;**8**(sup2):741-750

[28] Barbut S. Convenience breaded poultry meat products—New developments. Trends in Food Science and Technology. 2012;**26**(1):14-20

[29] Pasiakos SM, Agarwal S, Lieberman HR, Fulgoni VL III. Sources and amounts of animal, dairy, and plant protein intake of US adults in 2007-2010. Nutrients. 2015;**7**(8):7058-7069

[30] Ricke SC. Poultry Food Safety and Foodborne Illness. Elsevier; 2024

[31] Alali WQ, Hofacre CL. Preharvest food safety in broiler chicken production. Preharvest Food Safety. 1 Jul 2018:69-86

[32] Betiku E, Ogundipe TT, Kalapala T, Obe T. A mini-review on multi-hurdle

control of *Salmonella* along poultry production continuum. Animals. 2025;**15**(6):875

[33] Yue K, Cao Q-q, Shaukat A, Zhang C, Huang S-c. Insights into the evaluation, influential factors and improvement strategies for poultry meat quality: A review. npj Science of Food. 2024;**8**(1):62

[34] Banerjee DK, Das A, Thakur N, Talukder S, Das A, Sonowal J, et al. Factors affecting microbial growth in livestock products: A review. International Journal of Chemical Studies. 2019;**7**(3):4017-4022

[35] Liljebjelke KA, Hofacre CL, Liu T, White DG, Ayers S, Young S, et al. Vertical and horizontal transmission of *Salmonella* within integrated broiler production system. Foodbourne Pathogens and Disease. 2005;**2**(1):90-102

[36] Crespo R, Jeffrey J, Chin R, Senties-Cue G, Shivaprasad H. Phenotypic and genotypic characterization of *Salmonella* arizonae from an integrated Turkey operation. Avian Diseases. 2004;**48**(2):344-350

[37] Bailey J, Cox N, Berrang M. Hatchery-acquired *Salmonellae* in broiler chicks. Poultry Science. 1994;**73**(7):1153-1157

[38] Bailey J, Cox N, Craven S, Cosby D. Serotype tracking of *Salmonella* through integrated broiler chicken operations. Journal of Food Protection. 2002;**65**(5):742-745

[39] Oakley BB, Lillehoj HS, Kogut MH, Kim WK, Maurer JJ, Pedroso A, et al. The chicken gastrointestinal microbiome. FEMS Microbiology Letters. 2014;**360**(2):100-112

[40] De Reu K, Grijspeerdt K, Messens W, Heyndrickx M, Uyttendaele M, Debevere J, et al. Eggshell factors influencing eggshell penetration and whole egg contamination by different bacteria, including *Salmonella enteritidis*. International Journal of Food Microbiology. 2006;**112**(3):253-260

[41] Padron M. *Salmonella* Typhimurium penetration through the eggshell of hatching eggs. Avian Diseases. 1 Apr 1990:463-465

[42] Kopanic RJ Jr, Sheldon BW, Wright CG. Cockroaches as vectors of *Salmonella*: Laboratory and field trials. Journal of Food Protection. 1994;**57**(2):125-131

[43] Leffer AM, Kuttel J, Martins LM, Pedroso AC, Astolfi-Ferreira CS, Ferreira F, et al. Vectorial competence of larvae and adults of *Alphitobius diaperinus* in the transmission of *Salmonella* Enteritidis in poultry. Vector-Borne and Zoonotic Diseases. 2010;**10**(5):481-487

[44] Sparagano O. Control of poultry mites: Where do we stand? Experimental and Applied Acarology. 2009;**48**(1):1-2

[45] Davies RH, Hinton MH. *Salmonella* in Animal Feed. CABI Publishing; 2000

[46] Kallapura G, Hernandez-Velasco X, Pumford NR, Bielke LR, Hargis BM, Tellez G. Evaluation of respiratory route as a viable portal of entry for *Salmonella* in poultry. Veterinary Medicine: Research and Reports. 14 Aug 2014:59-73

[47] Zwe YH, Tang VCY, Aung KT, Gutiérrez RA, Ng LC, Yuk H-G. Prevalence, sequence types, antibiotic resistance and, *gyrA* mutations of *Salmonella* isolated from retail fresh chicken meat in Singapore. Food Control. 2018;**90**:233-240

[48] Gorman R, Bloomfield S, Adley CC. A study of cross-contamination

of food-borne pathogens in the domestic kitchen in the Republic of Ireland. International Journal of Food Microbiology. 2002;**76**(1-2):143-150

[49] Carrasco E, Morales-Rueda A, García-Gimeno RM. Cross-contamination and recontamination by *Salmonella* in foods: A review. Food Research International. 2012;**45**(2):545-556

[50] De Boer E, Hahné M. Cross-contamination with *Campylobacter jejuni* and *Salmonella* spp. from raw chicken products during food preparation. Journal of Food Protection. 1990;**53**(12):1067-1068

[51] Baéza E. Characteristics of processed poultry products. World's Poultry Science Journal. 2020;**76**(4):719-741

[52] Hobbs JL, Warshawsky B, Maki A, Zittermann S, Murphy A, Majury A, et al. Nuggets of wisdom: *Salmonella* Enteritidis outbreaks and the case for new rules on uncooked frozen processed chicken. Journal of Food Protection. 2017;**80**(4):703-709

[53] Morton V, Kearney A, Coleman S, Viswanathan M, Chau K, Orr A, et al. Outbreaks of *Salmonella* illness associated with frozen raw breaded chicken products in Canada, 2015-2019. Epidemiology and Infection. 2019;**147**:e254

[54] Bucher O, Holley R, Ahmed R, Tabor H, Nadon C, Ng L, et al. Occurrence and characterization of *Salmonella* from chicken nuggets, strips, and pelleted broiler feed. Journal of Food Protection. 2007;**70**(10):2251-2258

[55] Eglezos S, Dykes GA, Huang B, Fegan N, Stuttard E. Bacteriological profile of raw, frozen chicken nuggets. Journal of Food Protection. 2008;**71**(3):613-615

[56] Meneses R, Teixeira P. Marination as a hurdle to microbial pathogens and spoilers in poultry meat products: A brief review. Applied Sciences. 2022;**12**(22):11774

[57] Park NY, Hong SH, Yoon KS. Effects of commercial marinade seasoning and a natural blend of cultured sugar and vinegar on *Campylobacter jejuni* and *Salmonella* Typhimurium and the texture of chicken breasts. Poultry Science. 2014;**93**(3):719-727

[58] Dominguez SA, Schaffner DW. Survival of *Salmonella* in processed chicken products during frozen storage. Journal of Food Protection. 2009;**72**(10):2088-2092

[59] Willis C, Jørgensen F, Cawthraw S, Aird H, Lai S, Kesby M, et al. A survey of *Salmonella*, *Escherichia coli*, and antimicrobial resistance in frozen, part-cooked, breaded, or battered chicken products on retail sale in the UK. Journal of Applied Microbiology. 2023;**134**(5):lxad093

[60] Khan AS, Georges K, Rahaman S, Abdela W, Adesiyun AA. Prevalence and serotypes of *Salmonella* spp. on chickens sold at retail outlets in Trinidad. PLoS ONE. 2018;**13**(8):e0202108

[61] Beterams A, Tolksdorf T, Martin A, Stingl K, Bandick N, Reich F. Change of *Campylobacter*, *Escherichia coli* and *Salmonella* counts in packaged broiler breast meat stored under modified atmosphere and vacuum conditions at 4 and 10 C based on cultural and molecular biological quantification. Food Control. 2023;**145**:109337

[62] Centers for Disease Control and Prevention. Reports of Selected

Salmonella Outbreak Investigations. Atlanta, GA: Centers for Disease Control and Prevention; 2019. p. 3

[63] Authority EFS. The European Union one health 2018 zoonoses report. EFSA Journal. 2019;**17**(12):e05926

[64] Ferrari RG, Rosario DK, Cunha-Neto A, Mano SB, Figueiredo EE, Conte-Junior CA. Worldwide epidemiology of *Salmonella* serovars in animal-based foods: A meta-analysis. Applied and Environmental Microbiology. 2019;**85**(14):e00591-19

[65] Humphrey T, Baskerville A, Mawer S, Rowe B, Hopper S. *Salmonella* Enteritidis phage type 4 from the contents of intact eggs: A study involving naturally infected hens. Epidemiology and Infection. 1989;**103**(3):415-423

[66] Humphrey T, Whitehead A, Gawler A, Henley A, Rowe B. Numbers of *Salmonella* Enteritidis in the contents of naturally contaminated hens' eggs. Epidemiology and Infection. 1991;**106**(3):489-496

[67] Gantois I, Ducatelle R, Pasmans F, Haesebrouck F, Gast R, Humphrey TJ, et al. Mechanisms of egg contamination by *Salmonella* Enteritidis. FEMS Microbiology Reviews. 2009;**33**(4):718-738

[68] Kang H, Loui C, Clavijo R, Riley L, Lu S. Survival characteristics of *Salmonella* enterica serovar Enteritidis in chicken egg albumen. Epidemiology and Infection. 2006;**134**(5):967-976

[69] Schoeni JL, Glass KA, McDermott JL, Wong AC. Growth and penetration of *Salmonella* Enteritidis, *Salmonella* Heidelberg and *Salmonella* Typhimurium in eggs. International Journal of Food Microbiology. 1995;**24**(3):385-396

[70] Bradshaw JG, Shah DB, Forney E, Madden JM. Growth of *Salmonella* Enteritidis in yolk of shell eggs from normal and seropositive hens. Journal of Food Protection. 1990;**53**(12):1033-1036

[71] Ebel E, Schlosser W. Estimating the annual fraction of eggs contaminated with *Salmonella* Enteritidis in the United States. International Journal of Food Microbiology. 2000;**61**(1):51-62

[72] Centers for Disease Control and Prevention. Outbreaks of *Salmonella* Infections Linked to Backyard Poultry. Atlanta, GA: Centers for Disease Control and Prevention. Available from: https://wwwcdcgov/salmonella/backyardpoultry-05-20/indexhtml; [Accessed: June 19, 2021]2020

[73] Zielicka-Hardy A, Zarowna D, Szych J, Madajczak G, Sadkowska-Todys M. Ensuring safety of home-produced eggs to control salmonellosis in Poland: Lessons from an outbreak in September 2011. Eurosurveillance. 2012;**17**(47):20319

[74] Manning J, Gole V, Chousalkar K. Screening for *Salmonella* in backyard chickens. Preventive Veterinary Medicine. 2015;**120**(2):241-245

[75] Andreoletti O, Budka H, Buncic S, Collins JD, Griffin J, Hald T, et al. Scientific opinion on a quantitative estimate of the public health impact of setting a new target for the reduction of *Salmonella* in laying hens. EFSA Journal. 2010;**8**(4)

[76] Howard ZR, O'Bryan CA, Crandall PG, Ricke SC. *Salmonella* Enteritidis in shell eggs: Current issues and prospects for control. Food Research International. 2012;**45**(2):755-764

[77] Mumma GA, Griffin PM, Meltzer MI, Braden CR, Tauxe RV.

Egg quality assurance programs and egg-associated *Salmonella* Enteritidis infections, United States. Emerging Infectious Diseases. 2004;**10**(10):1782

[78] Brown LG, Hoover ER, Selman CA, Coleman E, Rogers HS. Outbreak characteristics associated with identification of contributing factors to foodborne illness outbreaks. Epidemiology and Infection. 2017;**145**(11):2254-2262

[79] Jones AK, Cross P, Burton M, Millman C, O'Brien SJ, Rigby D. Estimating the prevalence of food risk increasing behaviours in UK kitchens. PLoS ONE. 2017;**12**(6):e0175816

[80] Cardoso MJ, Nicolau AI, Borda D, Nielsen L, Maia RL, Møretrø T, et al. *Salmonella* in eggs: From shopping to consumption—A review providing an evidence-based analysis of risk factors. Comprehensive Reviews in Food Science and Food Safety. 2021;**20**(3):2716-2741

[81] Costerton JW, Lewandowski Z, Caldwell DE, Korber DR, Lappin-Scott HM. Microbial biofilms. Annual Review of Microbiology. 1995

[82] Milanov D, Ljubojević D, Čabarkapa I, Karabasil N, Velhner M. Biofilm as risk factor for *Salmonella* contamination in various stages of poultry production. European Poultry Science. 2017;**81**:1-14

[83] Ramesh N, Joseph S, Carr L, Douglass L, Wheaton F. Evaluation of chemical disinfectants for the elimination of *Salmonella* biofilms from poultry transport containers. Poultry Science. 2002;**81**(6):904-910

[84] Gradel K, Jørgensen JC, Andersen J, Corry J. Laboratory heating studies with *Salmonella* spp. and *Escherichia coli* in organic matter, with a view to decontamination of poultry houses. Journal of Applied Microbiology. 2003;**94**(5):919-928

[85] Paniel N, Noguer T. Detection of *Salmonella* in food matrices, from conventional methods to recent aptamer-sensing technologies. Foods. 2019;**8**(9):371

[86] Lee SI, Kim SA, Park SH, Ricke SC. Molecular and new-generation techniques for rapid detection of foodborne pathogens and characterization of microbial communities in poultry meat. In: Food Safety in Poultry Meat Production. Springer; 2019. pp. 235-260

[87] Basler C, Nguyen T-A, Anderson TC, Hancock T, Behravesh CB. Outbreaks of human *Salmonella* infections associated with live poultry, United States, 1990-2014. Emerging Infectious Diseases. 2016;**22**(10):1705

[88] Centers for Disease Control and Prevention. *Salmonella* Outbreak Linked to Ground Turkey. 2022

[89] Centers for Disease Control and Prevention. *Salmonella* Outbreak Linked to Raw Frozen Breaded Stuffed Chicken Products. 2021

[90] Centers for Disease Control and Prevention. *Salmonella* Outbreaks Linked to Backyard Poultry. 2021. p. 1

[91] Punchihewage-Don AJ, Hawkins J, Adnan AM, Hashem F, Parveen S. The outbreaks and prevalence of antimicrobial resistant *Salmonella* in poultry in the United States: An overview. Heliyon. 2022;**8**(11)

[92] US Food and Drug Administration. NARMS Integrated Report 2014. Laurel, MD. Available from: https://www.fda.gov/AnimalVeterinary/SafetyHealth/AntimicrobialResistance/

NationalAntimicrobialResistance MonitoringSystem/ucm059103.htm: US Food and Drug Administration, Department of Health and Human Services; 2017

[93] Folster JP, Pecic G, Rickert R, Taylor J, Zhao S, Fedorka-Cray P, et al. Characterization of multidrug-resistant *Salmonella enterica* serovar Heidelberg from a ground Turkey-associated outbreak in the United States in 2011. Antimicrobial Agents and Chemotherapy. 2012;**56**(6):3465-3466

[94] Gokulan K, Khare S, Rooney AW, Han J, Lynne AM, Foley SL. Impact of plasmids, including those encodingVirB4/D4 type IV secretion systems, on *Salmonella enterica* serovar Heidelberg virulence in macrophages and epithelial cells. PLoS ONE. 2013;**8**(10):e77866

[95] Multistate C, editor. Outbreak of Human *Salmonella* Altona and *Salmonella* Johannesburg Infections Linked to Chicks and Ducklings (Final Update). CDC; 2011

[96] Green AL, Klos R, Kirkpatrick J, Douris A, Cosgrove S, Miller B, et al. Multi-drug resistant *Salmonella* Hadar infections associated with Turkey burger consumption. Food Protection Trends. 2014;**34**(3)

[97] Lin C-S, Lu T-L, Chen Y-A, Yu H-Y, Wu C-Y, Yang W-Y. Safety of bivalent live attenuated *Salmonella* vaccine and its protection against bacterial shedding and tissue invasion in layers challenged with *Salmonella*. Poultry Science. 2022;**101**(7):101943

[98] Huberman YD, Caballero-García M, Rojas R, Ascanio S, Olmos LH, Malena R, et al. The efficacy of a trivalent inactivated *Salmonella* vaccine combined with the live *S.* Gallinarum 9R vaccine in young layers after experimental infections with *S.* Enteritidis, *S.* Typhimurium, and *S.* Infantis. Vaccines. 2022;**10**(7):1113

[99] El Hage R, El Hage J, Snini SP, Ammoun I, Touma J, Rachid R, et al. The detection of potential native probiotics *Lactobacillus* spp. against *Salmonella* Enteritidis, *Salmonella* Infantis, and *Salmonella* Kentucky ST198 of Lebanese chicken origin. Antibiotics. 2022;**11**(9):1147

[100] Ovuru KF, Izah SC, Ogidi OI, Imarhiagbe O, Ogwu MC. Slaughterhouse facilities in developing nations: Sanitation and hygiene practices, microbial contaminants and sustainable management system. Food Science and Biotechnology. 2024;**33**(3):519-537

[101] Buncic S, Sofos J. Interventions to control *Salmonella* contamination during poultry, cattle and pig slaughter. Food Research International. 2012;**45**(2):641-655

[102] Northcutt J, Smith D, Musgrove M, Ingram K, Hinton A Jr. Microbiological impact of spray washing broiler carcasses using different chlorine concentrations and water temperatures. Poultry Science. 2005;**84**(10):1648-1652

[103] National Advisory Committee on Microbiological Criteria for Foods. Generic HACCP application in broiler slaughter and processing. Journal of Food Protection. 1997;**60**(5):579-604

[104] Kandeepan G, Tahseen A. Modified atmosphere packaging (map) of meat and meat products: A review. Journal of Packaging Technology and Research. 2022;**6**(3):137-148

[105] Popa EE, Miteluț AC, Râpă M, Popescu PA, Drăghici MC,

Geicu-Cristea M, et al. Antimicrobial active packaging containing nisin for preservation of products of animal origin: An overview. Foods. 2022;**11**(23):3820

[106] Rajendran S, Mallikarjunan PK, O'Neill E. High pressure processing for raw meat in combination with other treatments: A review. Journal of Food Processing and Preservation. 2022;**46**(10):e16049

[107] Singer RS. *Salmonella* Framework for Raw Poultry Products Critical Review January 17, 2025. 2025

[108] OIE. Prevention, Detection and Control of *Salmonella* in Poultry. Office International des Epizooties Paris; 2019

[109] Montoro-Dasi L, Lorenzo-Rebenaque L, Marco-Fuertes A, Vega S, Marin C. Holistic strategies to control *Salmonella* Infantis: An emerging challenge in the European broiler sector. Microorganisms. 2023;**11**(7):1765

[110] Neelawala RN, Edison LK, Kariyawasam S. Pre-harvest non-typhoidal *Salmonella* control strategies in commercial layer chickens. Animals. 2024;**14**(24):3578

[111] Redmond EC, Griffith CJ. Consumer food handling in the home: A review of food safety studies. Journal of Food Protection. 2003;**66**(1):130-161

[112] Rao M, Klappholz A, Tamber S. Effectiveness of preparation practices on the inactivation of *Salmonella* enterica serovar Enteritidis in frozen breaded chicken strips. Journal of Food Protection. 2020;**83**(8):1289-1295

[113] Kosa KM, Cates SC, Bradley S, Chambers IE, Godwin S. Consumer-reported handling of raw poultry products at home: Results from a national survey. Journal of Food Protection. 2015;**78**(1):180-186

[114] Kosa K, Cates S, Bradley S, Godwin S, Chambers E IV, Ricketts J, et al. Food thermometer usage among consumers who cook raw poultry. Journal of Food Protection. 2014;**77**(Suppl A):138

[115] Inguglia ES, Song Z, Kerry JP, O'Sullivan MG, Hamill RM. Addressing clean label trends in commercial meat processing: Strategies, challenges and insights from consumer perspectives. Foods. 2023;**12**(10):2062

[116] Medeiros LC, Hillers VN, Kendall PA, Mason A. Food safety education: What should we be teaching to consumers? Journal of Nutrition Education. 2001;**33**(2):108-113

[117] Bass SB, Brajuha J, Kelly PJ, D'Avanzo P, Lambertini E, Nordhagen S, et al. Changing behavior, attitudes, and beliefs about food safety: A scoping review of interventions across the world and implications for empowering consumers. Foodborne Pathogens and Disease. 2022;**19**(1):19-30

[118] Volkova V, Wills R, Hubbard S, Magee D, Byrd J, Bailey R. Risk factors associated with detection of *Salmonella* in broiler litter at the time of new flock placement. Zoonoses and Public Health. 2011;**58**(3):158-168

[119] Meher MM, Sharif MA, Al BA. Seroprevalence of *Salmonella* spp. infection in different types of poultry and biosecurity measures associated with salmonellosis. International Journal of Agriculture Environment and Food Sciences. 2022;**6**(4):557-567

[120] Pourabedin M, Guan L, Zhao X. Xylo-oligosaccharides and virginiamycin differentially modulate gut microbial

composition in chickens. Microbiome. 2015;**3**:1-12

[121] Morelli L, Capurso L. FAO/WHO guidelines on probiotics: 10 years later. Journal of Clinical Gastroenterology. 2012;**46**:S1-S2

[122] Khan S, Chousalkar KK. *Salmonella* Typhimurium infection disrupts but continuous feeding of *Bacillus* based probiotic restores gut microbiota in infected hens. Journal of Animal Science and Biotechnology. 2020;**11**:1-16

[123] Henriques A, Sereno R, Almeida A. Reducing *Salmonella* horizontal transmission during egg incubation by phage therapy. Foodborne Pathogens and Disease. 2013;**10**(8):718-722

[124] Nabil NM, Tawakol MM, Hassan HM. Assessing the impact of bacteriophages in the treatment of *Salmonella* in broiler chickens. Infection Ecology & Epidemiology. 2018;**8**(1):1539056

[125] Malik D. Bacteriophage encapsulation using spray drying for phage therapy. Current Issues Molecular Biology. 2021

[126] Jia S, McWhorter AR, Andrews DM, Underwood GJ, Chousalkar KK. Challenges in vaccinating layer hens against *Salmonella* typhimurium. Vaccine. 2020;**8**(4):696

[127] Shin H, La T-M, Lee H-J, Kim T, Song S-u, Park E, et al. Evaluation of immune responses and protective efficacy of a novel live attenuated *Salmonella* Enteritidis vaccine candidate in chickens. Vaccine. 2022;**10**(9):1405

[128] Shaji S, Selvaraj RK, Shanmugasundaram R. *Salmonella* infection in poultry: A review on the pathogen and control strategies. Microorganisms. 2023;**11**(11):2814

[129] Crouch CF, Nell T, Reijnders M, Donkers T, Pugh C, Patel A, et al. Safety and efficacy of a novel inactivated trivalent *Salmonella enterica* vaccine in chickens. Vaccine. 2020;**38**(43):6741-6750

[130] Li Q, Ren J, Xian H, Yin C, Yuan Y, Li Y, et al. rOmpF and OMVs as efficient subunit vaccines against *Salmonella enterica* serovar Enteritidis infections in poultry farms. Vaccine. 2020;**38**(45):7094-7099

[131] Okamura M, Matsumoto W, Seike F, Tanaka Y, Teratani C, Tozuka M, et al. Efficacy of soluble recombinant FliC protein from *Salmonella enterica* serovar Enteritidis as a potential vaccine candidate against homologous challenge in chickens. Avian Diseases. 2012;**56**(2):354-358

[132] Jiang X, Chu C, Wang Z, Gu J, Hong Y, Li Q, et al. Preclinical evaluation of OMVs as potential vaccine candidates against *Salmonella enterica* serovar Enteritidis infection. Frontiers in Cellular and Infection Microbiology. 2022;**12**:1037607

[133] Staff AO. Risk Assessments for *Salmonella* in Eggs and Broiler Chickens: Interpretative Summary. World Health Organization; 2002

[134] Marmion M, Macori G, Ferone M, Whyte P, Scannell A. Survive and thrive: Control mechanisms that facilitate bacterial adaptation to survive manufacturing-related stress. International Journal of Food Microbiology. 2022;**368**:109612

[135] de Mesquita Souza Saraiva M, Lim K, do Monte DF, Givisiez PE, Alves LB, de Freitas Neto OC, et al. Antimicrobial resistance in the globalized food chain: A One Health perspective applied to the poultry industry. Brazilian Journal of Microbiology. Mar 2022;**53**(1):465-486

Chapter 5

Non-Typhoidal *Salmonella*: Decoding Mechanisms for Effective Disease Control

Adishi Ranjan, Aayushi Patel, Andrew Wolfram, Seetha Lakshmi and Taseen S. Desin

Abstract

Non-typhoidal *Salmonella* (NTS) species are a leading cause of foodborne illnesses globally, with significant morbidity in both developed and developing countries. This chapter explores the molecular basis of NTS pathogenesis, highlighting the roles of *Salmonella* pathogenicity islands (SPIs), Type III Secretion Systems (T3SS), and host-pathogen interactions. Emphasis is placed on the molecular epidemiology of prevalent serotypes such as *Salmonella* Typhimurium (*S.* Typhimurium) and *S.* Enteritidis, as well as their adaptive mechanisms in various food and environmental niches. The chapter also reviews emerging multidrug-resistant strains and discusses current strategies for controlling transmission through improved diagnostics, public health surveillance, and food safety interventions.

Keywords: non-typhoidal *salmonella* (NTS), type 3 secretion systems, pathogenicity islands, multidrug resistance (MDR), control, prevention

1. Introduction

1.1 Overview and prevalence

Salmonella enterica (*S. enterica*) is a Gram-negative facultative intracellular bacterial pathogen that is a member of the *Enterobacteriaceae* family [1]. *S. enterica* consists of more than 2600 serovars of which *S. enterica* subspecies *enterica* is composed of serovars like *S.* Typhi that are host-adapted serovars restricted to humans, while other serovars like *S.* Enteritidis and *S.* Typhimurium are broad host range serovars affecting multiple species [2]. Typically, *S.* Typhi human infections are characterized by typhoid fever and invasive disease [3]. However, non-typhoidal *Salmonella* (NTS) species are one of the leading causes of self-limiting bacterial gastrointestinal disease in humans [4]. Interestingly, NTS species have been associated with invasive disease (iNTS) in sub-Saharan Africa that manifests as bacteremia leading to a case fatality rate of 20.6% [5]. The consumption of contaminated poultry products has been attributed to serve as the main source of human NTS infections, though fresh produce has emerged as a significant contributor in recent outbreaks [6]. NTS human infections result in an estimated annual global burden of 93.8 million cases leading to 155,000 deaths [7]. According to the Centers for Disease Control and Prevention (CDC), NTS species are responsible for an estimated 1.35 million cases of Salmonellosis annually, making them the second most common cause of foodborne illness [8]. This accounts for approximately 19,336 hospitalizations, a loss of 17,000 quality-adjusted life years (QALYs), and an estimated USD $3.3 billion in annual healthcare costs and productivity losses [9]. Additionally, NTS serotypes Enteritidis and Typhimurium are the predominant serotypes associated with human infections in Africa, Asia, Europe, Latin America and the Caribbean, and in North America [10].

1.2 Sources and transmission

According to data from the CDC's National Outbreak Reporting System (NORS), 3115 outbreaks were reported from 2009 to 2023 in the United States that were

State	Number of *Salmonella* outbreaks (2009–2023)
Minnesota	324
Texas	356
Ohio	363
Illinois	378
California	416
New York	436
Pennsylvania	436

Table 1.
States with the highest number of Salmonella *outbreaks (2009–2023) reported by the National Outbreak Reporting System (CDC) [11].*

Outbreak source	Date	Cases	Hospitalizations	Deaths	Number of states
Charcuterie Meats	Jan 2024	104	27	0	33
Fresh Basil	Apr 2024	36	4	0	14
Backyard Poultry	May 2024	470	125	1	48
Pet Bearded Dragons	Jun 2024	26	10	0	13
Cucumbers	Jun 2024	551	155	0	34
Small Turtles	Aug 2024	63	28	0	22
Eggs	Sep 2024	93	34	0	12
Geckos	Feb 2025	49	4	0	27
Cucumbers	May 2025	69	29	0	21
Eggs	Jun 2025	34	38	1	10
Backyard Poultry	Jun 2025	187	42	1	42
Pistachio Cream	Jun 2025	4	1	0	2
Frozen Sprouted Beans	July 2025	11	4	0	10

Table 2.
Recent Salmonella *outbreaks in the U.S. reported by the CDC [13].*

attributed to NTS species, resulting in 70,458 illnesses, 11,866 hospitalizations and 108 deaths [11]. Moreover, states with the highest number of *Salmonella* outbreaks in the U.S. over the 14-year period included Minnesota (324), Texas (356), Ohio (363), Illinois (378), California (416), New York (436) and Pennsylvania (436) (**Table 1**) [11]. Over 75% of the described outbreaks were linked to foodborne transmission, originating from a variety of sources including seeded vegetables, chicken, fruits, pork, beef, eggs and other produce [12]. Additionally, recent *Salmonella* outbreaks in 2024-2025 (**Table 2**) include those that are associated with charcuterie meats, fresh basil, backyard poultry, pet bearded dragons, cucumbers, small turtles, eggs, geckos, cucumbers, pistachio cream, and frozen sprouted beans [13], implying that *Salmonella* surveillance and control are critical steps in ensuring a safer food supply that will ultimately lead to lower human infections [14–17]. Taken together, the need to further understand molecular mechanisms of *Salmonella* pathogenesis and virulence are vital since the incidence of NTS and iNTS, along with the associated Multidrug Resistance (MDR) are on the rise [18].

2. Molecular virulence factors

2.1 Introduction to NTS virulence mechanisms

NTS serovars, such as *S.* Typhimurium and *S.* Enteritidis, are major causes of foodborne illness worldwide, typically resulting in self-limiting gastroenteritis in immunocompetent hosts. However, in vulnerable populations, including infants, the elderly, and the immunocompromised, NTS can breach the intestinal barrier, resulting in invasive bloodstream infections [5]. The pathogenesis of NTS involves a coordinated series of virulence mechanisms that enable intestinal invasion, immune evasion, and intracellular survival [19]. These mechanisms are largely encoded on chromosomal *Salmonella* pathogenicity islands (SPIs) and serovar-specific virulence plasmids, which together orchestrate the bacterium's ability to colonize, invade, and persist within the host [20, 21]. Therefore, an in-depth understanding of molecular virulence determinants is crucial for developing effective strategies aimed at controlling this pathogen.

2.2 *Salmonella* pathogenicity islands

SPI are clusters of genes coding for virulence factors [22]. These operons are distinct from other regions of DNA due to their high content of Cytosine and Guanine [23]. The proteins coded for within these operons facilitate the survival of the bacterium within various hosts and environments. Twenty-four such SPIs have been identified in *Salmonella* spp. (**Table 3**), with SPI-1 and SPI-2 having been the best characterized [24].

SPI-1 is conserved across all *Salmonella* spp. [25]. It encodes a Type 3 Secretion System (T3SS) and several effector molecules which are then translocated into host cells via a needle-like injectisome to help invade the epithelium [26]. Major effector molecules include SipA, which plays a role in actin rearrangement in host cells, SipB and SipC, which help with adhesion to epithelial cells [26, 27]. AvrA helps prevent apoptosis of infected macrophages to allow bacterial dissemination in the host [28].

SPI-2 is found in *Salmonella enterica* that is primarily expressed once the bacterium is inside the host cell within a membrane bound vacuole [29]. It encodes a

SPI	Presence	Key genetic features
SPI-1	Present in all *S. enterica* serovars	Encodes T3SS-1 and invasion effectors (Sip, Sop, Hil regulators); mediates epithelial invasion
SPI-2	Present in *S. enterica*	Encodes T3SS-2 and intracellular survival effectors (Sse, Ssp); essential for survival in macrophages
SPI-3	Variable	Encodes *mgtABC* (Mg^{2+} transport) and *MisL* adhesin; contributes to gut colonization and survival in macrophages
SPI-4	Variable	Encodes Type I Secretion System (T1SS) and non-fimbrial adhesin
SPI-5	Variable	Encodes effector proteins co-regulated and secreted by T3SS-1/T3SS-2 (e.g., PipB, SopB) which modulate inflammation
SPI-6	Strain-specific	Encodes Type VI Secretion System (T6SS); involved in bacterial competition and virulence in intestinal environment
SPI-7	Absent in NTS	Encodes Vi capsule genes of *S.* Typhi
SPI-8, 15	Absent in most NTS	Found in *S.* Typhi
SPI-9, 14	Variable among NTS	Encode adhesive or metabolic traits; contribute modestly to systemic colonization in some serovars
SPI-10, 11, 12	Variable	Implicated in oxidative stress survival
SPI 13	*S.* Enteritidis	Macrophage uptake
SPI-16–24	Mostly lineage-specific	Represent accessory or prophage-like islands; may encode serovar-specific T6SS

Table 3.
Summary of the Salmonella *pathogenicity islands and their key effectors [24].*

second T3SS (T3SS-2), as well as secreted effector proteins which play a major role in bacterial survival and replication within host cells [30]. These effector proteins help regulate the positioning of the *Salmonella*-containing vacuole (SCV), modulating cytoskeletal rearrangements, inhibiting the host inflammatory cytokines and delaying macrophage cytotoxicity [31].

2.3 Type 3 secretion systems

The T3SS is a nanomachine complex found in a number of Gram-negative bacteria, including *Yersinia, Shigella,* Enteropathogenic *Escherichia coli,* and *Salmonella* [32]. These injectisomes allow bacterial effector proteins to be injected directly into host cells [33]. Typically, the T3SS is comprised of a translocon, tip complex, needle, basal body, and cytoplasmic ATPase complex [34]. The basal body is made up of two rings, which help anchor the complex to the inner and outer membrane of the bacterial cell wall [35], while the needle is a hollow polymeric rod that allows effector proteins to be secreted [36]. Additionally, the tip complex, on top of the needle, interacts with the host cells [37] and the translocon forms pores in the host cell membrane to allow for the passage of effector molecules [38]. *Salmonella enterica* possesses two distinct T3SS, with T3SS-1 being functional during the initial invasion stage and T3SS-2 aiding in intracellular survival within the SCV. However, both are structurally analogous (**Table 4**) [39].

Component	T3SS-1	T3SS-2	Function
ATPase	InvC	SsaN	Powers secretion
Needle protein	PrgI	SsaG	Forms the central needle structure
Inner membrane ring	PrgH, PrgK	SsaV, SsaJ, SsaK	Anchors apparatus in membrane
Outer membrane ring	InvG	SsaC	Creates export pore
Tip proteins	SipD	SseB, SseC, SseD	Forms translocon & host contact
Effector chaperones	SicA, InvB	SscA, SsaE, SseA	Stabilize & deliver effectors

Table 4.
Comparing T3SS-1 and T3SS-2 and the homology of the proteins.

2.4 Virulence plasmids

Virulence plasmids are extrachromosomal DNA elements found in certain serovars of *Salmonella,* including Choleraesuis, Dublin, Enteritidis, and Typhimurium [40]. The gene products of these plasmids are not essential for the initial phase of intestinal colonization; however, they have been implicated in enhancing the intracellular survival of the pathogen [41]. All serovars with the plasmid carry the highly conserved, *spvRABCD* locus, yet the plasmid itself varies in size across the different serovars, ranging anywhere from 50 to 95 kb [42]. *spvR* encodes a transcriptional regulator that upregulates the operon in the intracellular environment while SpvA downregulates the operon. Taken together, the action of both of these regulators allows for tight transcriptional control [43]. SpvB is a cytotoxin with ADP-ribosyltransferase activity that blocks host cell actin polymerization, aiding in the proliferation of *Salmonella* within macrophages [44]. SpvC blocks MAP kinase signaling pathways and has potent anti-inflammatory effects shown to promote bacterial dissemination in murine models [45]. Additionally, SpvD is a hydrolase that inhibits the NF-κB pathway [46].

3. *Salmonella* antibiotic resistance

3.1 Introduction and scope of the problem

Antibiotic-resistant *Salmonella* presents a pressing challenge in modern food safety and public health [47]. The magnitude of this problem is significant and on the rise. In 2013, the CDC published an antibiotic resistance threat list, which categorized both NTS and *Salmonella* Typhi as "serious threats". That year, drug-resistant NTS and *Salmonella* Typhi accounted for 100,000 (8% of total NTS infections that year; 3% resistant to ciprofloxacin, 3% resistant to ceftriaxone; 5% resistant to 5 or more antibiotics) and 3800 (67% of total infections that year; 67% resistant to ciprofloxacin) infections across the United States, respectively [48]. In just 6 years, these numbers rose to approximately 255,000 (9% resistance to ciprofloxacin in 2020) and 6000 (85% resistance to ciprofloxacin in 2020), respectively [49].

However, the global nature of this crisis extends far beyond American borders. In Bangladesh, the combined prevalence of *Salmonella* in livestock and poultry is 37%, with tetracycline showing the highest resistance rates at 81% [50]. In China, a comprehensive meta-analysis revealed that the pooled prevalence of *Salmonella* isolated from pork was 17%, with high antibiotic resistance rates observed for tetracycline (68%), sulfisoxazole (65%), ampicillin (43%), streptomycin (42%), and sulfamethoxazole (42%) [51]. **Table 5** displays an increasing trend in *Salmonella* antibiotic resistance to commonly used antibiotics in humans, livestock, poultry, and pork.

3.2 Origins and drivers of resistance

The development of antibiotic resistance in *Salmonella* is linked to agricultural practices and the extensive use of antibiotics in food animal production. The global demand for high-value animal protein has driven countries to adopt highly profitable production systems that rely heavily on antimicrobials to maintain productivity and animal health [53]. The intensive nature of modern animal production systems has created conditions that promote the development and dissemination of antimicrobial resistance. Antibiotics are routinely employed in livestock operations for multiple purposes: growth promotion, prophylactic prevention of disease, therapeutic treatment of infections, and metaphylactic control of disease outbreaks [54]. The scale of this usage is remarkable, with previous studies indicating that antibiotic consumption for non-therapeutic purposes in poultry, swine, and cattle outweighs human antibiotic use by several-fold [55]. This approach, while economically advantageous, has contributed significantly to the antimicrobial resistance crisis.

3.3 Molecular mechanisms of resistance

The molecular basis of antibiotic resistance in *Salmonella* is complex and multifaceted. Resistance is primarily driven by horizontal gene transfer through plasmids, integrons, and transposons [56]. These mobile genetic elements carry genes that encode various antibiotic resistance mechanisms, including efflux pumps, mutations in target genes, and the production of β-lactamases such as TEM, SHV, and CTX-M [57–59]. Major resistance genes have been identified in various *Salmonella* serovars isolated from the food supply, including resistance to β-lactams, extended-spectrum β-lactams, fluoroquinolones, aminoglycosides, tetracyclines, and chloramphenicol [60]. This expanding resistance profile makes treatment of *Salmonella* increasingly challenging by limiting therapeutic options for clinicians. A particularly concerning aspect of *Salmonella* resistance is the role of biofilm formation. Biofilm production is a major factor contributing to antibiotic resistance, as it can directly and indirectly shield bacteria from the effects of antibiotic action [61]. *Salmonella* can form biofilms on both abiotic and biotic surfaces, including gallstones and epithelial cells, leading to persistent infections and reinfection cycles [61]. The minimum inhibitory concentration (MIC) and minimum bactericidal concentration (MBC) values of antibiotics can increase 100- to 1000-fold due to biofilm formation, making treatment significantly more difficult [62].

3.4 Environmental reservoirs and transmission pathways

The environmental dimension of antibiotic resistance adds another layer of complexity to the *Salmonella* resistance problem. Environmental microorganisms serve as excellent sources of antimicrobial resistance genes, collectively termed the 'environmental resistome' [63]. This resistome plays a critical role in transferring antimicrobial resistance to pathogenic microorganisms and directly affects human health

DOI: http://dx.doi.org/10.5772/intechopen.1012641

Year	Country	Source	Serovar	Antibiotic(s)	Resistance rate	Reference
2013	United States	Humans	*Salmonella* Typhi	Ciprofloxacin	67%	[48]
2013	United States	Humans	NTS	Ceftriaxone	3%	[48]
2013	United States	Humans	NTS	Ciprofloxacin	3%	[48]
2013	United States	Humans	NTS	5 or more antibiotics	5%	[48]
2003	United States	Poultry	*S.* Heidelberg	5 or more antibiotics	67%	[52]
2003	United States	Poultry	*S.* Kentucky	5 or more antibiotics	54%	[52]
2003	United States	Poultry	NTS	3 or more antibiotics	20%	[52]
2003	United States	Poultry	NTS	Streptomycin	30.9%	[52]
2003	United States	Poultry	NTS	Sullfadimethoxine	20.9%	[52]
2003	United States	Poultry	NTS	Tetracycline	13.9%	[52]
2003	United States	Poultry	NTS	Gentamicin	5.1%	[52]
2003	United States	Poultry	NTS	Trimethoprim - sulfamethoxazole	8.6%	[52]
2020	United States	Humans	NTS	ciprofloxacin	9%	[49]
2020	United States	Humans	*Salmonella* Typhi	Ciprofloxacin	85%	[49]
2000–2022	China	Pork	NTS	Tetracycline	68%	[51]
2000–2022	China	Pork	NTS	Sulfioxazole	65%	[51]
2000–2022	China	Pork	NTS	Ampicillin	43%	[51]
2000–2022	China	Pork	NTS	Streptomycin	42%	[51]
2000–2022	China	Pork	NTS	Sulfamethoxazole	42%	[51]
2000–2022	Bangladesh	Livestock + Poultry	NTS	Tetracycline	81%	[50]
2000–2022	Bangladesh	Livestock + Poultry	NTS	Oxtetracycline	52%	[50]

Year	Country	Source	Serovar	Antibiotic(s)	Resistance rate	Reference
2000–2022	Bangladesh	Livestock + Poultry	NTS	Doxycycline	51%	[50]
2000–2022	Bangladesh	Livestock + Poultry	NTS	Sulfamethoxazole/Trimethoprim	42%	[50]
2000–2022	Bangladesh	Livestock + Poultry	NTS	Ciprofloxacin	20%	[50]
2000–2022	Bangladesh	Livestock + Poultry	NTS	Gentamycin	11%	[50]
2000–2022	Bangladesh	Livestock + Poultry	NTS	Neomycin	4%	[50]

All studies reported a growing trend of antibiotic resistance over time.

Table 5.
Reported Salmonella *resistance rates to antibiotics.*

by entering the food chain [63]. The transmission pathways for antibiotic-resistant *Salmonella* are numerous and interconnected. Lactic acid bacteria have been identified as carriers of resistance genes that may serve as reservoirs for enteropathogenic bacteria like *Salmonella* [54]. Erythromycin, vancomycin, and tetracycline resistance genes have been identified in lactic acid-producing bacteria isolated from fermented dairy products, sausages, and raw meat products, including poultry, beef, and pork [64]. Foodborne pathogens can enter farms through various sources, including contaminated water, fecal matter, personnel, equipment, vehicles, insects, rodents and pets [65]. The movement of portable equipment and vehicles can act as vectors for carrying pathogens to farms and slaughterhouses [66]. Furthermore, antibiotic-resistant bacteria spread through washing systems, floors, flush systems, and holding pens, potentially ending up in animal carcasses [67]. Particularly noteworthy is the finding that antibiotic-resistant pathogens such as *S.* Typhimurium have been recovered from swine and poultry housed in antibiotic-free production systems, highlighting the important role of 'environmental ressistomes' in spreading resistance [63, 68].

3.5 Regional variations and emerging patterns

The prevalence and patterns of NTS antibiotic resistance show significant regional variations, reflecting differences in agricultural practices, regulatory frameworks, and surveillance systems. Studies from commercial poultry farms revealed concerning levels of multidrug resistance with *Salmonella* isolates showing resistance to streptomycin (30.9%), gentamicin (12.6%), sulfadimethoxine (20.9%), tetracycline (13.9%), and trimethoprim-sulfamethoxazole combination (8.6%) [52]. Among these isolates, 20% were resistant to three or more antibiotics, while 67% of *S.* Heidelberg and 54% of *S.* Kentucky isolates showed resistance to five or more antibiotics [52]. The global trends in *Salmonella* antibiotic resistance are concerning. As previously stated, the United States experienced a doubling in the prevalence of drug-resistant *Salmonella* in less than 6 years [48, 49]. Similarly, in Bangladesh, meta-analysis revealed a significant positive correlation between *Salmonella* prevalence and time [50]. A recent Chinese meta-analysis also detected a growing trend in *Salmonella* prevalence in pork over time [51].

3.6 Public health implications and future outlook

The threat of antibiotic resistance has far-reaching consequences for human health and well-being, including increased healthcare costs, productivity losses, and higher susceptibility to other serious illnesses [69]. The long-term projections are sobering. If no further political measures are taken to address the spread of antimicrobial resistance, it is expected to cause over 10 million deaths per year by 2050, exceeding cancer-related deaths [70]. Given the limited pipeline for new antimicrobials, expert management of currently available drugs has become critical [53]. In response to these challenges, the World Health Organization (WHO), in collaboration with the Food and Agriculture Organization (FAO) and the World Organization for Animal Health (WOAH), has declared antimicrobial resistance an issue of global concern that requires a holistic and multi-sectoral approach [53]. Regulatory agencies have begun implementing measures to address agricultural antibiotic use, with the Food and Drug Administration (FDA) issuing rules to phase out antibiotics from agriculture and require veterinary oversight for therapeutic antibiotic use in food animals and poultry [71].

3.7 Alternative approaches and future directions

The recognition of this growing antibiotic resistance challenge has sparked interest in alternative approaches to pathogen control. Alternatives such as probiotics, prebiotics, and phytobiotics are being tested against drug-resistant pathogens due to their broad spectrum of antimicrobial activity [72]. Ideally, these alternatives should be non-toxic, not result in residue buildup, palatable to animals, stable in the gut, capable of augmenting beneficial flora, and effective at inactivating harmful pathogens [54]. Another promising method of combating antimicrobial resistance is the development of efflux pump inhibitors. Inhibition of efflux systems and interruption of biofilm formation may reverse antibiotic resistance in bacteria and potentiate antibiotic efficiency [61]. Additionally, research has shown that the ability of pathogens to form biofilms decreases after deletion of various efflux pumps, including *acrD, acrEF, emrAB, macAB, mdfA, mdsABC, mdtBC, mdtK, and tolC* from *Salmonella enterica* serovars [73].

3.8 Challenges with antibiotic resistance

The challenge of antibiotic-resistant *Salmonella* in the food supply represents a complex, multifaceted problem that requires coordinated global action. Extensive use of antibiotics, combined with an intricate web of environmental reservoirs and transmission pathways, has created a situation where resistance continues to grow despite various control efforts. The regional variations, yet consistent global rise in resistance patterns, underscore the need for global action tailored to local agricultural practices and regulatory environments. Moving forward, success in controlling *Salmonella* antibiotic resistance will depend on the implementation of comprehensive strategies that combine judicious antibiotic use, enhanced surveillance systems, improved biosecurity measures, and the development of effective alternatives to traditional antimicrobials [60]. The stakes continue to rise as the continued spread of resistance threatens food supply safety and the effectiveness of antimicrobial therapy for treating human infections.

4. Controlling NTS through prevention, surveillance and vaccination

4.1 Surveillance and control

Strong surveillance and response systems are key to managing NTS infections around the world. In the U.S., the CDC created a PulseNet network that helps track and respond to foodborne outbreaks by connecting public health labs across the country. Using tools like whole genome sequencing (WGS) and pulsed-field gel electrophoresis (PFGE), PulseNet can quickly identify clusters of related *Salmonella* cases. This allows health officials to trace sources, contain outbreaks, and implement targeted public health measures more efficiently [74, 75].

Working alongside PulseNet is FoodNet, the Foodborne Diseases Active Surveillance Network, which tracks trends in foodborne illnesses at selected sites across the country. FoodNet plays a key role in providing incidence data, assessing the impact of food safety policies, and detecting emerging pathogens. Together, PulseNet and FoodNet form the foundation of the country's efforts to detect, investigate, and reduce NTS infections, shaping national public health strategies [76].

Globally, similar surveillance efforts are driven by international collaborations like the European Food Safety Authority (EFSA) and the European Centre for Disease Prevention and Control (ECDC). Together, they publish annual zoonosis reports that track *Salmonella* in food, animals, and humans across Europe [77].

Food recalls are one of the most visible outcomes of strong surveillance systems. When NTS is detected in food products, agencies such as the FDA or USDA can issue recalls to stop the spread and protect public health [78]. Early detection and a coordinated response play a key role in limiting the impact of outbreaks. Beyond removing contaminated products from the market, these recalls also highlight gaps in food safety practices, which encourage broader improvements across the supply chain [79].

Another key part of controlling NTS infections is the careful use of antibiotics, especially for high-risk groups. While most NTS infections resolve on their own, treatment is recommended for people who are more vulnerable, such as infants, older adults, and those with weakened immune systems [80]. Antibiotics may be needed when symptoms include high fever, persistent diarrhea, bacteremia, or other signs of a more serious, invasive infection [81]. However, the growing issue of antimicrobial resistance is a major concern. Multidrug-resistant *Salmonella* strains are on the rise, complicating treatment and reinforcing the need for responsible antibiotic use [82, 83].

4.2 Prevention and vaccination

Public education and strong food safety regulations play crucial roles in preventing NTS infections. Key strategies include promoting safe food handling and hygiene practices, as well as enforcing regulations throughout the food production and distribution process. These efforts aim to reduce infection rates by limiting the spread of the bacteria at both the individual and system-wide levels [84].

Public education focused on hygiene and safe food preparation serves as a critical method of primary prevention by reducing the risk of the initial NTS infection and is represented as the bottom tier of the prevention pyramid in **Figure 1**. Handwashing is a simple but powerful tool, especially given the zoonotic and fecal-oral transmission of *Salmonella*. The CDC's *Life is Better with Clean Hands and #KeepHandsClean* campaigns are a national effort aimed at raising awareness about the importance of handwashing at homes and in public settings [84]. By offering clear, practical guidance on when and how to wash hands, the campaign helps prevent not just *Salmonella* infections but a range of gastrointestinal and respiratory illnesses, including but not limited to Norovirus, *Shigella*, *E. coli*, Rotavirus, Influenza, and the common cold [85, 86].

In addition to hand hygiene, everyday food safety practices at the consumer level are essential for preventing NTS infections. These include cooking poultry and eggs to safe internal temperatures, avoiding raw or undercooked high-risk foods, preventing cross-contamination in the kitchen, and keeping perishable items properly refrigerated, consistent with CDC's Clean, Separate, Cook & Chill framework [87]. Moreover, public health messages promoting these habits are disseminated via public service announcements, food packaging labels, and local education efforts.

Educational campaigns in schools, childcare centers, and food service establishments build lifelong food safety habits. CDC partners with initiatives such as the Partnership for Food Safety Education's Fight BAC! campaign, which delivers consumer-focused food safety education grounded in the "Clean–Separate–Cook–Chill" model [88]. Additionally, educational campaigns in schools, childcare centers, and food service establishments play a vital role in building lifelong food safety habits. In food service environments, certification programs are often required by local

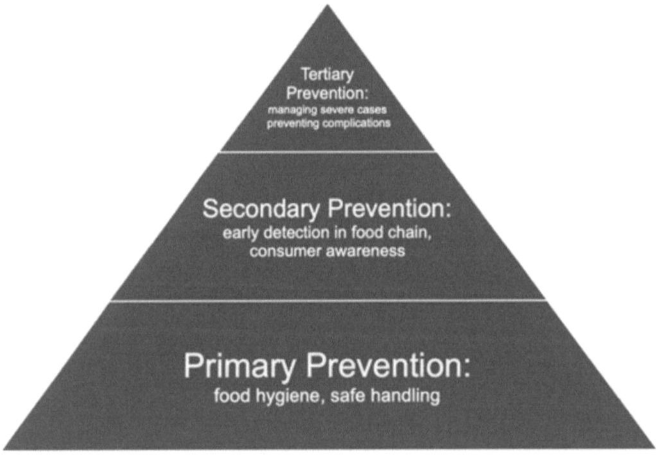

Figure 1.
This diagram illustrates primary prevention, secondary prevention and tertiary prevention for NTS infections.

health departments to educate workers on *Salmonella* prevention, safe food handling, and sanitation [89]. These training courses emphasize the importance of personal hygiene, proper temperature control, and thorough cleaning practices, all of which are critical for interrupting the transmission of foodborne pathogens. Numerous studies confirm that following basic hygiene and food-handling guidelines significantly lowers the risk of NTS transmission [86, 89].

At the policy level, food safety regulations are the foundation of large-scale prevention efforts. One of the most important frameworks is the Hazard Analysis Critical Control Point (HACCP) system. Originally developed for NASA's space food program, HACCP has since become a global standard and is now required across many parts of the food industry. The system focuses on controlling critical points in the production process where contamination is most likely to occur. HACCP is widely implemented in poultry processing facilities to reduce microbial contamination and maintain consistent safety standards [90, 91]. In addition, agencies like the USDA and FDA enforce strict *Salmonella* performance standards in meat and poultry processing facilities. Regular inspections are carried out to monitor compliance, including microbial testing, audits of sanitation practices, and reviews of facility HACCP plans. The use of WGS data from surveillance programs like PulseNet, help these efforts by enabling regulators to trace outbreaks and quickly identify weaknesses in food safety systems [76, 87]. In summary, secondary prevention efforts, as depicted by the second tier of the prevention pyramid in **Figure 1**, includes early detection and rapid response measures such as PulseNet's WGS surveillance, HACCP reviews, and public health education to detect and address risks early.

Finally, tertiary prevention, represented as the third tier of the prevention pyramid in **Figure 1**, focuses on the clinical management of NTS infections and the prevention of complications such as dehydration, bacteremia, endovascular infections, and osteomyelitis. It also includes antimicrobial stewardship, particularly in cases involving multidrug-resistant strains (as discussed in the *Salmonella Antibiotic Resistance* section of this chapter). Tertiary prevention is especially important for high-risk populations, including immunocompromised individuals, such as those with HIV, and groups at risk for invasive infection, such as neonates under 3 months of age, adults over 50 with suspected atherosclerosis, and individuals with cardiac conditions, immunosuppression, or significant joint disease [86].

Vaccine name/ platform	Antigen(s)/serovar COVERAGE	Vaccine type/ platform	Stage of development	Key immunogenicity Features	Target population/ indication	References
iNTS-GMMA	*S.* Typhimurium, *S.* Enteritidis O-antigen	GMMA (outer membrane vesicles)	Phase I/II clinical trials	Broad bactericidal antibody response	Infants/children in sub-Saharan Africa	[94]
iNTS-TCV (iNTS-GMMA + TYPHIBEV)	*S.* Typhimurium, *S.* Enteritidis, *S.* Typhi	GMMA + Vi conjugate (combination)	Phase I/II clinical trials	Broad coverage, including typhoid	Infants/children in endemic regions	[94]
OSP-rT2544 Glycoconjugate	*S.* Typhimurium OSP + rT2544 (outer membrane protein); cross-protection vs. *S.* Enteritidis, *S.* Typhi, *S.* Paratyphi	Glycoconjugate subunit	Preclinical (animal models)	High IgG/IgA, memory B/T cell response	Broad, including children	[95]
Multi-epitope (OmpA/OmpD/Stn)	*S.* Typhimurium, *S.* Enteritidis (OmpA, OmpD, enterotoxin)	Multi-epitope peptide (in silico)	In silico validation	Predicted strong T/B cell, cytokine response	Not yet defined	[96]
Multi-epitope (OmpA/C/F, fliC adjuvant)	*S.* Kentucky (OmpA, OmpC, OmpF), fliC from *S.* Typhimurium	Multi-epitope peptide (in silico)	In silico validation	Predicted high population coverage, robust immune response	Not yet defined	[97]
Pan-*Salmonella* Multi-epitope	CsgA (curlin major subunit A, conserved)	Multi-epitope peptide (in silico)	In silico validation	Predicted broad protection, robust immune response	Not yet defined	[98]
Live-attenuated NTS vaccines	*S. Typhimurium*, *S. Enteritidis* (various)	Live-attenuated bacterial	Preclinical/early clinical	Cellular and humoral immunity	Not yet defined	[92, 99]

Table 6.
NTS human vaccine candidates under development.

Efforts to control NTS through public education and food safety regulations have led to important progress. However, these measures alone are unlikely to achieve sustained global control, especially in high-burden areas like sub-Saharan Africa where vulnerable populations face the greatest risk [92]. In these regions, vaccination is emerging as a critical next step, particularly given the growing threat of multidrug-resistant NTS strains that limit treatment options [93]. Although no NTS vaccine has been officially licensed for human use as of 2025, several promising candidates are moving through the development pipeline [93]. These vaccines, their serovar coverage and stage of development are shown in **Table 6**.

Beyond these, innovative strategies such as subunit vaccines targeting conserved proteins like InvH, small extracellular vesicle-based platforms, and antigens identified through reverse vaccinology have demonstrated encouraging results in animal models [100, 101]. While these approaches show promise, they face practical hurdles including limited strain coverage, high production costs, and the challenge of integrating new vaccines into existing immunization programs. Addressing these barriers will be essential to ensure that future NTS vaccines are both effective and accessible where they are needed most.

Acknowledgements

We thank the University of Central Florida College of Medicine Department of Medical Education for their gracious support.

Conflict of interest

The authors declare no conflict of interest.

DOI: http://dx.doi.org/10.5772/intechopen.1012641

Author details

Adishi Ranjan[1], Aayushi Patel[2], Andrew Wolfram[2], Seetha Lakshmi[3] and Taseen S. Desin[3]*

1 College of Medicine, University of Central Florida, Orlando, FL, USA

2 Trinity School of Medicine, Trinity Medical Sciences University, Roswell, GA, USA

3 Department of Medical Education, College of Medicine, University of Central Florida, Orlando, FL, USA

*Address all correspondence to: taseen.desin@ucf.edu

References

[1] Holt JG, Krieg NR, Sneath PHA, Staley JT, Williams ST. Part 5. In: Holt JG, Krieg NR, Sneath PHA, Staley JT, Williams ST, editors. Bergey's Manual of Determinative Bacteriology. 9th ed. USA: Williams & Wilkins; 1994. p. 186

[2] Gal-Mor O. Persistent infection and long-term carriage of typhoidal and nontyphoidal Salmonellae. Clinical Microbiology Reviews. 2018;**32**(1):e00088-e00018. DOI: 10.1128/CMR.00088-18

[3] Dougan G, Baker S. Salmonella enterica serovar Typhi and the pathogenesis of typhoid fever. Annual Review of Microbiology. 2014;**68**:317-336. DOI: 10.1146/annurev-micro-091313-103739

[4] Haselbeck AH, Panzner U, Im J, Baker S, Meyer CG, Marks F. Current perspectives on invasive nontyphoidal Salmonella disease. Current Opinion in Infectious Diseases. 2017;**30**(5):498-503. DOI: 10.1097/QCO.0000000000000398

[5] Kumar G, Kumar S, Jangid H, Dutta J, Shidiki A. The rise of non-typhoidal Salmonella: An emerging global public health concern. Frontiers in Microbiology. 2025;**16**:1524287. DOI: 10.3389/fmicb.2025.1524287

[6] Hanning IB, Nutt JD, Ricke SC. Salmonellosis outbreaks in the United States due to fresh produce: Sources and potential intervention measures. Foodborne Pathogens and Disease. 2009;**6**(6):635-648. DOI: 10.1089/fpd.2008.0232

[7] Majowicz SE, Musto J, Scallan E, Angulo FJ, Kirk M, O'Brien SJ, et al. The global burden of nontyphoidal Salmonella gastroenteritis. Clinical Infectious Diseases: An Official Publication of the Infectious Diseases Society of America. 2010;**50**(6):882-889. DOI: 10.1086/650733

[8] Centers for Disease Control and Prevention (CDC). Available from: https://www.cdc.gov/salmonella/about/index.html [Accessed: August 4, 2025]

[9] Cummings PL, Sorvillo F, Kuo T. The burden of salmonellosis in the United States. In: Mahmoud BSM, editor. Salmonella - A Dangerous Foodborne Pathogen. London: InTech; 2012. DOI: 10.5772/28019. ISBN 978-953-307-782-6

[10] Galanis E, Lo Fo Wong DM, Patrick ME, Binsztein N, Cieslik A, Chalermchikit T, et al. Web-based surveillance and global Salmonella distribution, 2000-2002. Emerging Infectious Diseases. 2006;**12**(3):381-388. DOI: 10.3201/eid1205.050854

[11] Centers for Disease Control and Prevention (CDC). BEAM (Bacteria, Enterics, Ameba, and Mycotics) Dashboard. Atlanta, Georgia: U.S. Department of Health and Human Services. 2025. Available from: www.cdc.gov/ncezid/dfwed/BEAM-dashboard.html; [Accessed: August 4, 2025]

[12] Pires SM, Vieira AR, Hald T, Cole D. Source attribution of human salmonellosis: An overview of methods and estimates. Foodborne Pathogens and Disease. 2014;**11**(9):667-676. DOI: 10.1089/fpd.2014.1744

[13] Centers for Disease Control and Prevention (CDC). Available from: https://www.cdc.gov/salmonella/outbreaks/index.html#cc-widget-50d5 [Accessed: August 4, 2025]

[14] Ghunaim H, Desin TS. Potential impact of food safety vaccines on health care costs. Foodborne Pathogens and Disease. 2015;**12**(9):733-740. DOI: 10.1089/fpd.2014.1924

[15] Patel A, Wolfram A, Desin TS. Advancements in detection methods for Salmonella in food: A comprehensive review. Pathogens (Basel, Switzerland). 2024;**13**(12):1075. DOI: 10.3390/pathogens13121075

[16] Desin TS, Köster W, Potter AA. Salmonella vaccines in poultry: Past, present and future. Expert Review of Vaccines. 2013;**12**(1):87-96. DOI: 10.1586/erv.12.138

[17] Gast RK. Serotype-specific and serotype-independent strategies for preharvest control of food-borne Salmonella in poultry. Avian Diseases. 2007;**51**(4):817-828. DOI: 10.1637/8090-081807.1

[18] Sia CM, Pearson JS, Howden BP, Williamson DA, Ingle DJ. Salmonella pathogenicity islands in the genomic era. Trends in Microbiology. 2025;**33**(7):752-764. DOI: 10.1016/j.tim.2025.02.007

[19] Coombes BK, Coburn BA, Potter AA, Gomis S, Mirakhur K, Li Y, et al. Analysis of the contribution of Salmonella pathogenicity islands 1 and 2 to enteric disease progression using a novel bovine ileal loop model and a murine model of infectious enterocolitis. Infection and Immunity. 2005;**73**(11):7161-7169. DOI: 10.1128/IAI.73.11.7161-7169.2005

[20] Galán JE. Salmonella interactions with host cells: Type III secretion at work. Annual Review of Cell and Developmental Biology. 2001;**17**:53-86. DOI: 10.1146/annurev.cellbio.17.1.53

[21] Kuhle V, Hensel M. Cellular microbiology of intracellular Salmonella enterica: Functions of the type III secretion system encoded by Salmonella pathogenicity island 2. Cellular and Molecular Life Sciences: CMLS. 2004;**61**(22):2812-2826. DOI: 10.1007/s00018-004-4248-z

[22] Gal-Mor O, Finlay BB. Pathogenicity islands: A molecular toolbox for bacterial virulence. Cellular Microbiology. 2006;**8**(11):1707-1719

[23] Hacker J, Blum-Oehler G, Mühldorfer I, Tschäpe H. Pathogenicity islands of virulent bacteria: Structure, function and impact on microbial evolution. Molecular Microbiology. 1997;**23**(6):1089-1097

[24] Sia CM, Pearson JS, Howden BP, Williamson DA, Ingle DJ. Salmonella pathogenicity islands in the genomic era. Trends in Microbiology. 2025;**33**(7):752-764. Advance online publication. DOI: 10.1016/j.tim.2025.03.006

[25] Fookes M, Schroeder GN, Langridge GC, Blondel CJ, Mammina C, Connor TR, et al. Salmonella bongori provides insights into the evolution of the Salmonellae. PLoS Pathogens. 2011;**7**(8):e1002191

[26] Lara-Tejero M, Galán JE. Salmonella enterica serovar typhimurium pathogenicity island 1-encoded type III secretion system translocases mediate intimate attachment to nonphagocytic cells. Infection and Immunity. 2009;**77**(7):2635-2642

[27] Zhou D, Mooseker MS, Galán JE. Role of the S. typhimurium actin-binding protein SipA in bacterial internalization. Science. 1999;**283**(5410):2092-2095

[28] Wu H, Jones RM, Neish AS. The Salmonella effector AvrA mediates bacterial intracellular survival during

infection in vivo. Cellular Microbiology. 2012;**14**(1):28-39

[29] Garcia-del Portillo F, Zwick MB, Leung KY, Finlay BB. Salmonella induces the formation of filamentous structures containing lysosomal membrane glycoproteins in epithelial cells. Proceedings of the National Academy of Sciences. 1993;**90**(22):10544-10548

[30] Ochman H, Soncini FC, Solomon F, Groisman EA. Identification of a pathogenicity island required for Salmonella survival in host cells. Proceedings of the National Academy of Sciences. 1996;**93**(15):7800-7804. DOI: 10.1073/pnas.93.15.7800

[31] Figueira R, Holden DW. Functions of the Salmonella pathogenicity island 2 (SPI-2) type III secretion system effectors. Microbiology. 2012;**158**(5):1147-1161

[32] Notti RQ, Stebbins CE. The structure and function of type III secretion systems. Microbiology Spectrum. 2016;**4**(1):1-18. VMBF-0004-2015. DOI: 10.1128/microbiolspec.VMBF-0004-2015

[33] Lee CA. Type III secretion systems: Machines to deliver bacterial proteins into eukaryotic cells? Trends in Microbiology. 1997;**5**(4):148-156. DOI: 10.1016/S0966-842X(97)01029-9

[34] Büttner D. Protein export according to schedule: Architecture, assembly, and regulation of type III secretion systems from plant- and animal-pathogenic bacteria. Microbiology and Molecular Biology Reviews. 2012;**76**(2):262-310. DOI: 10.1128/MMBR.05017-11

[35] Costa TRD, Felisberto-Rodrigues C, Meir A, Prevost MS, Redzej A, Trokter M, et al. Secretion systems in gram-negative bacteria: Structural and mechanistic insights. Nature Reviews Microbiology. 2015;**13**:343-359. DOI: 10.1038/nrmicro3456

[36] Kimbrough TG, Miller SI. Contribution of Salmonella typhimurium type III secretion components to needle complex formation. Proceedings of the National Academy of Sciences. 2000;**97**(20):11008-11013. DOI: 10.1073/pnas.200209497

[37] Chatterjee S, Zhong D, Nordhues BA, Battaile KP, Lovell S, De Guzman RN. The crystal structures of the Salmonella type III secretion system tip protein SipD in complex with deoxycholate and chenodeoxycholate. Protein Science. 2010;**20**(1):75-86. DOI: 10.1002/pro.537

[38] Nikolaus T, Deiwick J, Rappl C, Freeman JA, Schröder W, Miller SI, et al. SseBCD proteins are secreted by the type III secretion system of Salmonella pathogenicity island 2 and function as a translocon. Journal of Bacteriology. 2001;**183**(20):6036-6045. DOI: 10.1128/JB.183.20.6036-6045.2001

[39] Han J, Aljahdali N, Zhao S, Tang H, Harbottle H, Hoffmann M, et al. Infection biology of Salmonella enterica. EcoSal Plus. 2024;**12**(1):eesp00012023. DOI: 10.1128/ecosalplus.esp-0001-2023

[40] Chu C, Chiu CH. Evolution of the virulence plasmids of non-typhoid Salmonella and its association with antimicrobial resistance. Microbes and Infection. 2006;**8**(7):1931-1936

[41] Gulig PA, Danbara H, Guiney DG, Lax AJ, Norel F, Rhen M. Molecular analysis of spv virulence genes of the Salmonella virulence plasmids. Molecular Microbiology. 1993;**7**(6):825-830

[42] Sengupta M, Austin S. Prevalence and significance of plasmid maintenance

functions in the virulence plasmids of pathogenic bacteria. Infection and Immunity. 2011;**79**(7):2502-2509

[43] Passaris I, Cambre A, Govers SK, Aertsen A, Michiels CW. Bimodal expression of the Salmonella typhimurium spv operon. Genetics. 2018;**210**(2):621-635

[44] Browne SH, Hasegawa O, Okamoto K. Identification of Salmonella SPI-2 secretion system components required for SpvB-mediated cytotoxicity in macrophages and virulence in mice. FEMS Immunology & Medical Microbiology. 2008;**52**(2):194-201

[45] Haneda T, Ishii Y, Shimizu H, Ohno A, Kurokawa M, Tateda K. Salmonella type III effector SpvC, a phosphothreonine lyase, contributes to reduction in inflammatory response during intestinal phase of infection. Cellular Microbiology. 2012;**14**(4):485-499

[46] Grabe GJ, Zhang Y, Przydacz M, Fiedler S, Wittchen M. The Salmonella effector SpvD is a cysteine hydrolase with a serovar-specific polymorphism influencing catalytic activity, suppression of immune responses, and bacterial virulence. Journal of Biological Chemistry. 2023;**291**(50):25853-25863

[47] Kumar R, Adeyemi NO, Chattaraj S, Alloun W, Thamarsha AKANWMRK, Anđelković S, et al. Antimicrobial resistance in Salmonella: One health perspective on global food safety challenges. Science in One Health. 2025;**4**:100117. DOI: 10.1016/j.soh.2025.100117

[48] Centers for Disease Control and Prevention (CDC). Antibiotic Resistance Threats in the United States. 2013. Available from: https://www.cdc.gov/antimicrobial-resistance/media/pdfs/ar-threats-2013-508.pdf

[49] COVID-19: U.S. Impact on Antimicrobial Resistance, Special Report 2022. National Center for Emerging and Zoonotic Infectious Diseases. 2022. Available from: https://www.cdc.gov/antimicrobial-resistance/media/pdfs/covid19-impact-report-508.pdf

[50] Ripon RK, Motahara U, Ahmed A, Devnath N, Mahua FA, Hashem RB, et al. Exploring the prevalence of antibiotic resistance patterns and drivers of antibiotics resistance of Salmonella in livestock and poultry-derived foods: A systematic review and meta-analysis in Bangladesh from 2000 to 2022. JAC-Antimicrobial Resistance. 2023;**5**(3):dlad059. DOI: 10.1093/jacamr/dlad059

[51] Shen W, Chen H, Geng J, Wu RA, Wang X, Ding T. Prevalence, serovar distribution, and antibiotic resistance of Salmonella spp. isolated from pork in China: A systematic review and meta-analysis. International Journal of Food Microbiology. 2022;**361**:109473. DOI: 10.1016/j.ijfoodmicro.2021.109473

[52] Liljebjelke KA, Hofacre CL, White DG, Ayers S, Lee MD, Maurer JJ. Diversity of antimicrobial resistance phenotypes in salmonella isolated from commercial poultry farms. Frontiers in Veterinary Science. 2017;**4**:96. DOI: 10.3389/fvets.2017.00096

[53] McCormick BP, Quiroga MP, Álvarez VE, Centrón D, Tittonell P. Antimicrobial resistance dissemination associated with intensive animal production practices in Argentina: A systematic review and meta-analysis. Revista Argentina de Microbiología. 2023;**55**(1):25-42. DOI: 10.1016/j.ram.2022.07.001

[54] Nair VT, Venkitanarayanan K, Kollanoor Johny A. Antibiotic-resistant Salmonella in the food supply and the potential role of antibiotic alternatives for control. Foods. 2018;7(10):167. DOI: 10.3390/foods7100167

[55] Chang Q, Wang W, Regev-Yochay G, Lipsitch M, Hanage WP. Antibiotics in agriculture and the risk to human health: How worried should we be? Evolutionary Applications. 2015;**8**(3):240-247. DOI: 10.1111/eva.12185

[56] Carattoli A. Plasmid-mediated antimicrobial resistance in Salmonella enterica. Current Issues in Molecular Biology. 2003;**5**:113-122

[57] Mulvey MR, Soule G, Boyd D, Demczuk W, Ahmed R, Multi-provincial Salmonella Typhimurium Case Control Study Group. Characterization of the first extended-spectrum beta-lactamase-producing Salmonella isolate identified in Canada. Journal of Clinical Microbiology. 2003;**41**(1):460-462. DOI: 10.1128/JCM.41.1.460-462.2003

[58] Tassios PT, Gazouli M, Tzelepi E, Milch H, Kozlova N, Sidorenko S, et al. Spread of a Salmonella typhimurium clone resistant to expanded-spectrum cephalosporins in three European countries. Journal of Clinical Microbiology. 1999;**37**(11):3774-3777. DOI: 10.1128/JCM.37.11.3774-3777.1999

[59] Villa L, Pezzella C, Tosini F, Visca P, Petrucca A, Carattoli A. Multiple-antibiotic resistance mediated by structurally related IncL/M plasmids carrying an extended-spectrum beta-lactamase gene and a class 1 integron. Antimicrobial Agents and Chemotherapy. 2000;**44**(10):2911-2914. DOI: 10.1128/AAC.44.10.2911-2914.2000

[60] Cheng G, Hao H, Xie S, Wang X, Dai M, Huang L, et al. Antibiotic alternatives: The substitution of antibiotics in animal husbandry? Frontiers in Microbiology. 2014;**5**:1-15. Article 217. DOI: 10.3389/fmicb.2014.00217

[61] Alenazy R. Antibiotic resistance in Salmonella: Targeting multidrug resistance by understanding efflux pumps, regulators, and the inhibitors. Journal of King Saud University - Science. 2022;**34**(7):102275. DOI: 10.1016/j.jksus.2022.102275

[62] Gonzalez-Escobedo G, Gunn JS. Identification of Salmonella enterica serovar typhimurium genes regulated during biofilm formation on cholesterol gallstone surfaces. Infection and Immunity. 2013;**81**(10):3770-3780. DOI: 10.1128/IAI.00647-13

[63] Wright GD. Antibiotic resistance in the environment: A link to the clinic? Current Opinion in Microbiology. 2010;**13**(5):589-594. DOI: 10.1016/j.mib.2010.08.005

[64] Mathur S, Singh R. Antibiotic resistance in food lactic acid bacteria—A review. International Journal of Food Microbiology. 2005;**105**(3):281-295. DOI: 10.1016/j.ijfoodmicro.2005.03.008

[65] McEwen SA, Fedorka-Cray PJ. Antimicrobial use and resistance in animals. Clinical Infectious Diseases. 2002;**34**(Suppl. 3):S93-S106. DOI: 10.1086/340246

[66] Heyndrickx M, Vandekerchove D, Herman L, Rollier I, Grijspeerdt K, De Zutter L. Routes for salmonella contamination of poultry meat: Epidemiological study from hatchery to slaughterhouse. Epidemiology and Infection. 2002;**129**(2):253-265. DOI: 10.1017/s0950268802007380

[67] Dorr PM, Tadesse DA, Zewde BM, Fry P, Thakur S, Gebreyes WA.

Longitudinal study of Salmonella dispersion and the role of environmental contamination in commercial swine production systems. Applied and Environmental Microbiology. 2009;**75**(6):1478-1486. DOI: 10.1128/AEM.01632-08

[68] Alali WQ, Thakur S, Berghaus RD, Martin MP, Gebreyes WA. Prevalence and distribution of Salmonella in organic and conventional broiler poultry farms. Foodborne Pathogens and Disease. 2010;**7**(11):1363-1371. DOI: 10.1089/fpd.2010.0566

[69] National Academies of Sciences, Engineering, and Medicine. The health and economic burden of resistance. In: Combating Antimicrobial Resistance and Protecting the Miracle of Modern Medicine. Washington, DC (USA): National Academies Press; 2021. Available from: https://www.ncbi.nlm.nih.gov/books/NBK577288/

[70] Murray CJL, Ikuta KS, Sharara F, Swetschinski L, Aguilar GR, Gray A, et al. Global burden of bacterial antimicrobial resistance in 2019: A systematic analysis. The Lancet. 2022;**399**(10325):629-655. DOI: 10.1016/S0140-6736(21)02724-0

[71] U.S. Food and Drug Administration. Timeline of FDA Action on Antimicrobial Resistance. 2024. Available from: https://www.fda.gov/animal-veterinary/antimicrobial-resistance/timeline-fda-action-antimicrobial-resistance

[72] Gupta R, Sharma S. Role of alternatives to antibiotics in mitigating the antimicrobial resistance crisis. The Indian Journal of Medical Research. 2022;**156**(3):464-477. DOI: 10.4103/ijmr.IJMR_3514_20

[73] Baugh S, Ekanayaka AS, Piddock LJV, Webber MA. Loss of or inhibition of all multidrug resistance efflux pumps of Salmonella enterica serovar typhimurium results in impaired ability to form a biofilm. Journal of Antimicrobial Chemotherapy. 2012;**67**(10):2409-2417. DOI: 10.1093/jac/dks228

[74] Kubota KA, Wolfgang WJ, Baker DJ, Boxrud D, Turner L, Trees E, et al. PulseNet and the changing paradigm of laboratory-based surveillance for foodborne diseases. Public Health Reports (Washington, D.C.: 1974). 2019;**134**(Suppl. 2):22S-28S. DOI: 10.1177/0033354919881650

[75] Ribot EM, Freeman M, Hise KB, Gerner-Smidt P. PulseNet: Entering the age of next-generation sequencing. Foodborne Pathogens and Disease. 2019;**16**(7):451-456. DOI: 10.1089/fpd.2019.2634

[76] Ehuwa O, Jaiswal AK, Jaiswal S. Salmonella, food safety and food handling practices. Foods (Basel, Switzerland). 2021;**10**(5):907. DOI: 10.3390/foods10050907

[77] European Food Safety Authority (EFSA), European Centre for Disease Prevention and Control (ECDC). The European Union one health 2023 zoonoses report. EFSA Journal. European Food Safety Authority. 2024;**22**(12):e9106. DOI: 10.2903/j.efsa.2024.9106

[78] Dey M, Mayo JA, Saville D, Wolyniak C, Klontz KC. Recalls of foods due to microbiological contamination classified by the U.S. Food and Drug Administration, fiscal years 2003 through 2011. Journal of Food Protection. 2013;**76**(6):932-938. DOI: 10.4315/0362-028X.JFP-12-464

[79] DeBeer J, Blickem ER, Rana YS, Baumgartel DM, Bell JW. An analysis of food recalls in the United States,

2002-2023. Journal of Food Protection. 2024;**87**(12):100378. DOI: 10.1016/j.jfp.2024.100378

[80] Tsai MH, Huang YC, Lin TY, Huang YL, Kuo CC, Chiu CH. Reappraisal of parenteral antimicrobial therapy for nontyphoidal Salmonella enteric infection in children. Clinical Microbiology and Infection: The Official Publication of the European Society of Clinical Microbiology and Infectious Diseases. 2011;**17**(2):300-305. DOI: 10.1111/j.1469-0691.2010.03230.x

[81] Tack B, Vanaenrode J, Verbakel JY, Toelen J, Jacobs J. Invasive non-typhoidal Salmonella infections in sub-Saharan Africa: A systematic review on antimicrobial resistance and treatment. BMC Medicine. 2020;**18**(1):212. DOI: 10.1186/s12916-020-01652-4

[82] Liu FC, Chang YJ, Chen CL, Yang HP, Lee CC, Chiu CH. Clinical features, antimicrobial resistance, and serogroups of nontyphoidal Salmonella isolated from infants less than 3 months old in the recent decade. The Pediatric Infectious Disease Journal. 2022;**41**(10):813-818. DOI: 10.1097/INF.0000000000003656

[83] Kariuki S, Gordon MA, Feasey N, Parry CM. Antimicrobial resistance and management of invasive Salmonella disease. Vaccine. 2015;**33**(Suppl. 3):C21-C29. DOI: 10.1016/j.vaccine.2015.03.102

[84] Centers for Disease Control and Prevention. Life Is Better with Clean Hands. USA: U.S. Department of Health & Human Services; n.d.. Available from: https://www.cdc.gov/clean-hands/lifeisbetterwithcleanhands/index.html [Accessed: August 2, 2025]

[85] Shane AL, Mody RK, Crump JA, Phillip T I, Steiner TS, Kotloff K, et al. Infectious Diseases Society of America clinical practice guidelines for the diagnosis and management of infectious diarrhea. Clinical Infectious Diseases. 2017;**65**(12):e45-e80. DOI: 10.1093/cid/cix669

[86] Aiello AE, Coulborn RM, Perez V, Larson EL. Effect of hand hygiene on infectious disease risk in the community setting: A meta-analysis. American Journal of Public Health. 2008;**98**(8):1372-1381. DOI: 10.2105/AJPH.2007.124610

[87] Centers for Disease Control and Prevention. Food Safety. U.S. Department of Health & Human Services. USA: CDC. Available from: https://www.cdc.gov/food-safety/index.html; n.d. [Accessed: August 2, 2025]

[88] Partnership for Food Safety Education. The Core Four Practices. Fight BAC! n.d. USA: CDC, USDA and FDA. Available from: https://fightbac.org/food-safety-basics/the-core-four-practices/ [Accessed: August 2, 2025]

[89] Losasso C, Cappa V, Cibin V, Mantovani C, Costa N, Faccio E, et al. Food safety and hygiene lessons in the primary school: Implications for risk-reduction behaviors. Foodborne Pathogens and Disease. 2014;**11**(1):68-74. DOI: 10.1089/fpd.2013.1598

[90] Williams MS, Ebel ED. Estimating changes in public health following implementation of hazard analysis and critical control point in the United States broiler slaughter industry. Foodborne Pathogens and Disease. 2012;**9**(1):59-67. DOI: 10.1089/fpd.2011.0951

[91] Herrera AG. The hazard analysis and critical control point system in food safety. Methods in Molecular Biology (Clifton, N.J.). 2004;**268**:235-280. DOI: 10.1385/1-59259-766-1:235

[92] Martin LB, Tack B, Marchello CS, Sikorski MJ, Owusu-Dabo E, Nyirenda T,

et al. Vaccine value profile for invasive non-typhoidal Salmonella disease. Vaccine. 2024;**42**(19S1):S101-S124. DOI: 10.1016/j.vaccine.2024.04.045

[93] Nazir J, Manzoor T, Saleem A, Gani U, Bhat SS, Khan S, et al. Combatting Salmonella: A focus on antimicrobial resistance and the need for effective vaccination. BMC Infectious Diseases. 2025;**25**(1):84. DOI: 10.1186/s12879-025-10478-5

[94] De Simone D, Pinto M, Aruta MG, Benincasa M, Carducci M, Di Benedetto R, et al. GMMA-based vaccine candidates against invasive nontyphoidal salmonellosis elicit bactericidal antibodies against a panel of epidemiologically relevant Salmonellae. Frontiers in Immunology. 2025;**16**:1610067. DOI: 10.3389/fimmu.2025.1610067

[95] Haldar R, Dhar A, Ganguli D, Chakraborty S, Pal A, Banik G, et al. A candidate glycoconjugate vaccine induces protective antibodies in the serum and intestinal secretions, antibody recall response and memory T cells and protects against both typhoidal and non-typhoidal salmonella serovars. Frontiers in Immunology. 2024;**14**:1304170. DOI: 10.3389/fimmu.2023.1304170

[96] Beikzadeh B. Immunoinformatics design of multi-epitope vaccine using OmpA, OmpD and enterotoxin against non-typhoidal salmonellosis. BMC Bioinformatics. 2023;**24**(1):63. DOI: 10.1186/s12859-023-05183-6

[97] Igomu EE, Mamman PH, Adamu J, Muhammad M, Woziri AO, Sugun MY, et al. Immunoinformatics design of a novel multiepitope vaccine candidate against non-typhoidal salmonellosis caused by Salmonella Kentucky using outer membrane proteins A, C, and F. PLoS One. 2025;**20**(1):e0306200. DOI: 10.1371/journal.pone.0306200

[98] Bhattacharjee A, Hosen MR, Lamisa AB, Ahammad I, Chowdhury ZM, Jamal TB, et al. An integrated comparative genomics, subtractive proteomics and immunoinformatics framework for the rational design of a Pan-Salmonella multi-epitope vaccine. PLoS One. 2024;**19**(7):e0292413. DOI: 10.1371/journal.pone.0292413

[99] Sears KT, Galen JE, Tennant SM. Advances in the development of Salmonella-based vaccine strategies for protection against salmonellosis in humans. Journal of Applied Microbiology. 2021;**131**(6):2640-2658. DOI: 10.1111/jam.15055

[100] Choudhury M, Borah P, Sarma HK, Deka D, Dutta R, Hazarika G, et al. Development of recombinant subunit vaccine targeting InvH protein of Salmonella Typhimurium and evaluation of its immunoprotective efficacy against salmonellosis. Brazilian Journal of Microbiology. 2023;**54**(4):3257-3264. DOI: 10.1007/s42770-023-01136-6

[101] Emerson LE, Bhimani S, Rainey AL, Maurelli AT, Ferraro MJ. Evaluating small extracellular vesicle-based vaccination across heterologous Salmonella strains isolated from wastewater. Infection and Immunity. 2025;**93**(2):e0048524. DOI: 10.1128/iai.00485-24

Chapter 6

Mechanistic Insights into *Salmonella* Infections in Livestock

Adedeji O. Adetunji, Heidi Price, Henrietta Owusu, Emmanuel Asiamah and Olumuyiwa Olarotimi

Abstract

Salmonella infection continues to pose a significant global challenge in livestock production systems, impacting animal health, productivity, and food safety. This chapter examines the mechanisms through which *Salmonella* causes disease in livestock, emphasizing proinflammatory cytokine responses and the dynamics of host-pathogen interactions that play a role in intestinal inflammation and septicemia. Furthermore, the chapter explores the role of antibiotics in mitigating Salmonellosis. With the growing restrictions on antibiotic use in animal feed due to concerns over antimicrobial resistance, there is a heightened focus on exploring natural alternatives with inherent immunomodulatory, antimicrobial, and antioxidant properties. This includes the potential of plant extracts and spray-dried plasma (SDP) as sustainable methods for managing Salmonellosis in livestock. The chapter identifies the key targets of *Salmonella* action and the therapeutic targets of bacteriostats. It wraps up by emphasizing the potential of plant extracts and SDP as alternatives to in-feed antibiotics.

Keywords: *Salmonella*, livestock, antibiotics, plant extracts, spray dried plasma

1. Introduction

Salmonella is a bacterial infection that poses significant public health risks and economic loss, primarily through foodborne transmission. While poultry products are the most common source, the pathogen can affect humans and other animals. *Salmonella* is classified into two species, *Salmonella enterica and Salmonella bongori*. Within *S. enterica* are six subspecies, including *enterica, salamae, arizonae, diarizonae, houtenae, and indica*. The bacterium primarily spreads via infected hosts and contaminated food, such as animal products like meat, milk, and eggs. Still, it can also persist in environmental sources such as water and soil [1–3]. It typically targets the digestive tract, triggering immune responses like increased spleen cellularity and leukocyte recruitment to limit systemic infection. Infection with *Salmonella* diverts resources from normal physiological functions, often resulting in slower growth, reduced reproductive performance, and higher mortality in affected animals [4]. Consequently, *Salmonella* poses a severe economic burden on the livestock industry. The ability of *Salmonella* to adhere to, invade, and replicate within host cells, all while evading immune surveillance, is a key factor in its pathogenicity in livestock. The evolution of these bacteria has led to the development of specialized secretion systems, notably the Type III Secretion Systems (T3SS), capable of injecting virulent factors into host cells. This process manipulates cellular functions and enhances bacterial survival [5–7]. The immune response of the host to infection, marked by inflammation and the release of cytokines, plays a dual role in eliminating pathogens and causing tissue damage, particularly within the gastrointestinal tract [8, 9]. Moreover, the widespread use of antibiotics in both veterinary and human medicine has accelerated the emergence of antibiotic-resistant *Salmonella* strains, complicating efforts to treat and control infections [10]. This chapter delves into the detailed processes through which *Salmonella* initiates infection in livestock, covering aspects from intestinal colonization to systemic spread. Furthermore, studies have shown the potential of plant extracts in modulating several biochemical and metabolic activities [11] due to their inherent bioactive compounds. Similarly, Spray dried plasma (SDP) containing defensins, transferrin, amino acids, growth factors, and enzymes [12] have been reported to improve livestock performance in the presence of Salmonella infection [13]. Therefore, understanding these mechanisms is essential for creating efficient prevention and control strategies in contemporary animal agriculture.

1.1 Livestock species affected by *Salmonella*

1.1.1 Poultry

Salmonella is a significant pathogen in poultry production, with *Salmonella* enteritidis being the most prevalent serovar. Colonization by this pathogen is influenced by several factors, including the bird's age, environmental stressors, health status, diet, antimicrobial use, and genetic background. Young chicks are particularly susceptible due to their immature gut microflora. For *Salmonella* to establish infection, it must first survive acidic barriers in the crop, proventriculus, and gizzard before successfully attaching to and invading the host's intestinal lining [14]. Infections result in significant economic losses for poultry producers, as energy is diverted from growth to immune defense. Horizontal transmission is common, increasing the risk of spread within flocks. Although antimicrobials are still widely used, growing concerns over antimicrobial resistance and consumer skepticism have prompted the search for alternatives. These include probiotics, vaccination programs, improved biosecurity and hygiene practices, and competitive exclusion products. Beyond its impact on poultry, *Salmonella* poses serious public health risks, particularly through contaminated eggs and undercooked poultry, making it one of the leading causes of human foodborne illness.

1.1.2 Sheep

While poultry is one of the primary livestock species associated with *Salmonella* enteritidis due to the contamination of its products, other animals, including sheep, swine, and cattle, have also been implicated. Notably, cases involving sheep date back as early as 1919 and continue to be reported today, with approximately 20–30 cases recorded annually in the UK [15]. In sheep, *Salmonella* infections are often associated with *Salmonella* enterica subspecies and various serovars. Because *Salmonella* is not strictly host-specific, infected individuals within a flock can introduce and spread the pathogen to others, primarily through contaminated water sources and oral contact

[16]. Outbreaks often increase during periods of drought, when sheep are confined to limited grazing areas that become heavily contaminated. Once ingested, the pathogen can lead to serious health issues. In pregnant ewes, *Salmonella abortusovis* infection may result in abortion, stillbirths, or high maternal mortality, whereas nonpregnant ewes often show mild symptoms or remain asymptomatic, typically with lower mortality rates [17]. Treatment usually involves isolation, antibiotic therapy, and vaccination. However, some vaccines may be ineffective, particularly in cases where the disease re-emerges years after an initial outbreak, suggesting a potential for latent or environmental persistence that complicates disease control [18]. Because *Salmonella* can be transmitted to humans through direct contact or contaminated meat and dairy products, managing infections in sheep remains a critical concern for public health and food safety.

1.1.3 Swine

Salmonella is a prevalent pathogen in swine, primarily affecting the intestinal tract and raising concerns over contaminated pork products and animal health. The most common serovars in pigs are *S. Choleraesuis* and *S. Typhimurium*, and they cause significant economic losses due to high mortality, growth retardation, and increased treatment costs [19]. Infected pigs often appear asymptomatic, but some may exhibit clinical signs such as cyanosis and dyspnea, particularly on the ears and other body parts. *S. Choleraesuis* is typically isolated from the lymph nodes, tonsils, colon, and cecal contents [20]. It can be transmitted horizontally and remain viable in feces for up to 2 months after excretion. In contrast, *S. Typhimurium* tends to be less fatal, with most infected pigs recovering fully. However, its environmental persistence is a concern. Some studies have shown that this serovar can survive in soil for extended periods, with evidence of *Salmonella* presence up to 50 months after the initial outbreak [21]. Due to this longevity, rigorous sanitation is essential to prevent recurring outbreaks, alongside vaccination, to reduce the pathogen's ability to colonize internal organs. Beyond animal health, *Salmonella* also impacts pork safety. In the United States, pork products are among the top three food categories associated with *Salmonella*-related illnesses [22]. As a result, continuous monitoring of the food production chain is vital to identify contamination points and prevent contaminated products from reaching the market.

1.1.4 Cattle

Salmonella is a significant pathogen in the cattle industry, particularly in the dairy sector, where it risks animal health and food safety. The most prevalent serotype found in dairy operations is *S. Dublin*. This serotype is often asymptomatic but is associated with severe clinical outcomes, including true bacteremia, sepsis, abortion, pneumonia, and high mortality rates [23]. Infected cattle shed the bacteria orally through feces, contributing to environmental contamination and herd-level transmission. *Salmonella* spread horizontally within cattle populations like other livestock species, especially under crowded or unsanitary conditions. Outbreaks in cattle can result in substantial economic losses due to treatment costs, decreased milk production, weight loss, reduced fertility, and premature culling of chronically infected animals. Subclinical infections can go unnoticed but still contribute to reduced productivity over time. Additionally, *Salmonella* poses a major zoonotic threat through contaminated beef and unpasteurized dairy products. Human infection can occur from consuming undercooked meat or raw milk, and S. Dublin is known for causing invasive, sometimes life-threatening illnesses in people, particularly in vulnerable populations [24]. Effective management strategies include fluid therapy, antimicrobial treatment, colloid administration, and isolation of infected animals to prevent further spread and support recovery. Like swine, cattle are another important livestock species affected by *Salmonella*, posing both animal health challenges and public health risks due to the potential for contaminated beef and dairy products.

2. *Salmonella* and host interaction

Salmonella functions as a facultative intracellular pathogen, utilizing a sophisticated set of virulence strategies to penetrate host tissues, circumvent immune defenses, and cause illness in livestock. The onset of the disease process occurs when *Salmonella* is consumed through contaminated feed, water, or environmental contact. Upon entering the host, *Salmonella* specifically targets the gastrointestinal (GI) tract, focusing on the ileum and colon, where it adheres to and invades the intestinal epithelium [1, 2].

2.1 Adhesion and invasion

The first stage of *Salmonella* infection is characterized by its attachment to the intestinal epithelium. This process is facilitated by fimbriae and outer membrane proteins that identify particular receptors on host enterocytes. Upon attachment, *Salmonella* employs a type III secretion system (T3SS-1), which is encoded by genes located on the *Salmonella* Pathogenicity Island 1 (SPI-1), to deliver effector proteins into host cells. The effectors influence the host cytoskeleton, leading to membrane ruffling and aiding in the internalization of bacteria [3–5].

2.2 Intracellular survival and replication

Following internalization, *Salmonella* exists within a specialized phagosome known as the *Salmonella*-containing vacuole (SCV). The pathogen employs a second type III secretion system (T3SS-2, encoded by SPI-2) to manipulate host cell processes, effectively inhibiting lysosomal fusion and allowing for its survival and replication within macrophages [5, 6]. This intracellular environment facilitates the systemic dissemination of *Salmonella*, especially in young or immunocompromised animals [2].

2.3 Inflammatory response and gut damage

Salmonella infection elicits a robust proinflammatory response. The identification of pathogen-associated molecular patterns (PAMPs), including lipopolysaccharide (LPS) and flagellin, by host Toll-like receptors (TLRs) triggers the activation of the NF-κB signaling pathway. The outcome is the secretion of cytokines including IL-1β, IL-6, IL-8, and TNF-α, which facilitate the recruitment of neutrophils and the process of inflammation [7, 8]. In livestock, this is frequently manifested as enteritis, diarrhea, and diminished nutrient absorption resulting from epithelial damage [25].

2.4 Systemic dissemination and septicemia

In critical instances, particularly in neonates or compromised animals, *Salmonella* has the potential to breach the intestinal barrier and infiltrate the bloodstream, leading to septicemia. The liver and spleen frequently serve as colonization sites in the context of systemic infection [1]. This stage is linked to elevated mortality rates, especially among calves and piglets [2].

3. Mechanisms by which *Salmonella* causes disease in livestock

In livestock, *Salmonella* infection causes malabsorption, inefficient feed utilization, anemia, and reduced growth rate. Overall, this infection causes significant changes to immune cells, intestinal colonization, and invasion of internal lymphoid organs such as the spleen. According to Adetunji et al., the proteome signature of the spleen of broiler chickens shows an increase in the abundance of lysosomal proteins and proteins involved in responding to cellular stress, such as antioxidants and misfolded proteins [4]. Following the establishment of *Salmonella* infection, proteins associated with oxidative stress and mediate glutathione metabolism increased in abundance. In contrast, PRDX6, MGST1, and GPX1, which are related to the regulation of oxidative stress and reactive oxygen species (ROS), were downregulated. However, lysosomal proteins involved in the degradation of antigenic proteins increased in abundance. In the presence of *Salmonella* infection, the NF-kappa-B signaling pathway was triggered, leading to the production of inflammatory cytokines (tumor necrosis factor-alpha (TNF-α), interleukin, and type 1 interferons (IFNs)) (**Figure 1**). In the same manner, *Salmonella* infection causes the downregulation of proteins involved in proper protein folding and protein folding quality control. ALDOC, TKTL1, ASS1, and ASL proteins also perform cellular redox homeostasis maintenance functions [4, 26]. In addition to increasing the production of cytokines, *Salmonella* infection causes an increase in the abundance of genes involved in redox homeostasis, increased autophagy of infected cells, and misfolded protein binding. This prompts an innate response to foreign pathogens, clearance of antigenic proteins and infected cells, and the triggering of gluconeogenesis to meet the high energy demands of fighting the infection. More so, *Salmonella* infection causes the downregulation of proteins involved in actin filament binding, RNA binding, and the cytoskeleton (**Table 1**). Consequently, this suggests that *Salmonella* infection causes a diversion of energy required for body metabolism and other developmental processes to potentiate disease resistance mechanisms. As a result, signs and symptoms such as inefficient feed utilization, anemia, and reduced growth rate are manifested in the animal.

3.1 Mechanism by which antibiotic mitigates *Salmonella* action in a diseased state

Antibiotics are used to improve livestock's health, wellbeing, and growth performance [27]. Notably, Bacitracin Methylene Disalicylate (BMD), a bacteriostat, is incorporated into the animal diet as a feed additive to enhance digestion and prevent *Salmonella* enteritidis (SE) colonization of the intestinal tract. Rather than eliminate the bacteria infection, BMD interferes with protein synthesis and bacterial cell wall synthesis, resulting in microbial cell rupture and death. BMD facilitates the increase in abundance of RNA binding proteins, spliceosome, peptidyl-prolyl cis-trans isomerase activity, protein transport, and cell adhesion. In the presence of *Salmonella* infection, acute phase response signaling and GP6 signaling pathway were inhibited, while the pathway for the inhibition of ARE-mediated mRNA degradation pathway was activated. BMD acts in a manner that suppresses the production of proinflammatory cytokines (IL4, IL6, and AGT), ensures the proper folding of proteins, and

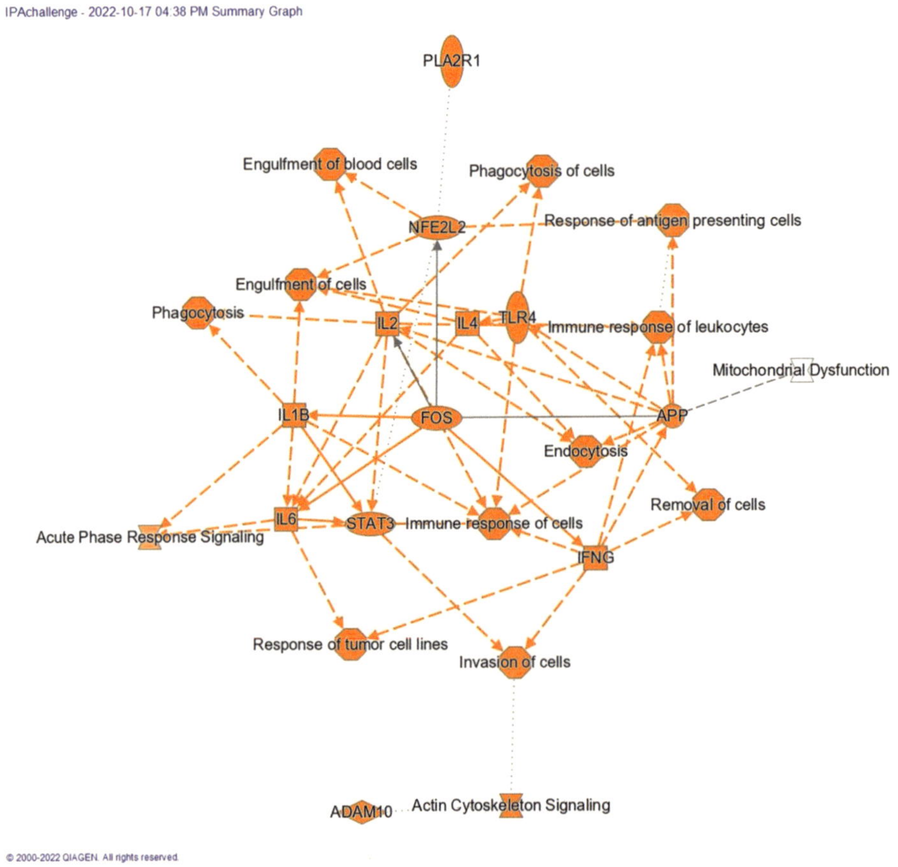

Figure 1.
IPA summary graph of the effect of Salmonella *showing an upregulation in inflammatory cytokines and associated proteins. In the figure, red represents upregulation. Direct and indirect interactions are indicated by solid, and dashed lines, respectively. The proteins interactions networks were generated using QIAGEN Inc. Ingenuity Pathway analysis, https://www.qiagenbioinformatics.com/products/ingenuity-pathway-analysis/ accessed on 17 October, 2022.*

promotes cell cycle progression. By so doing, it prevents the resultant effect of a cytokine storm in response to bacteria entry and selectively removes abnormally folded proteins through the Proteasome-mediated ubiquitin-dependent protein process rather than Lysosomal action or autophagy [28]. Notably, it also provides a source of amino acids useful in hypoxia conditions requiring gluconeogenesis, new protein synthesis, or ATP production (**Table 2**) [29].

3.2 Mechanism by which spray-dried plasma and plant extracts replace antibiotics in mitigating *Salmonella* infection

As discussed earlier, antibiotics (BMD) play two primary roles in mitigating *Salmonella* infection, and they include suppressing the production of cytokines and selective removal of infected cells while ensuring cell cycle progression. This is done to ensure the animal's day to day activities are not impacted despite the presence of infection. However, with the continuous clamor for the ban of antibiotic use in animal feed due to antimicrobial resistance issues, researchers have focused on the

Activities that occur during Salmonella infection	Decrease in protein abundance	Increase in protein abundance
ATP and oxygen demand increase		NPC2, CTSB, HSPA8, PPT1, CTSS, PRDX6, CTSS, PRDX6, FADD, CHUK
Lysosome degradation of antigenic proteins and infected cells		GOT1, ALDOC, ASS1, ASL, TKTL1, GOT2
RNA processing/cell cycle	HNRNPA3, NONO, MYH9, RPL19, MBNL1, ATXN2, EWSR1, FUBP1	

Table 1.
Increase and decrease in abundance of proteins during Salmonella *infection.*

Activities that occur during Salmonella infection with BMD treatment	Decrease in protein abundance	Increase in protein abundance
Regulation of actin cytoskeleton signaling induction of T cell activation, regulation of leucocyte migration	TM9SF2, MIA3, ITIH3	
Proinflammatory process facilitation	IL4, IL6, and AGT	
Components of fibrinogen	FN1, FGA, FGG, and FGB	
Proteasome-mediated ubiquitin-dependent protein process		RAD23A and RAD23B

Table 2.
Increase and decrease in abundance of proteins during Salmonella *infection with BMD treatment.*

use of natural compounds such as plant extracts and spray-dried plasma as alternatives to antibiotics. For instance, SDP has been reported to modulate immunological, biochemical, and metabolic activities due to its inherent immunoglobulins, peptides, amino acids, enzymes, and lipid constituents [12]. Histological studies have shown that by reducing intestinal inflammation, SDP may prevent the spread of bacteria or other antigens, hereby reducing immune activation locally [30]. Moreover, SDP supports intestinal health and broiler performance by creating a balance in intestinal microflora, thus improving digestibility [31, 32]. In addition, PCR studies show that SDP supplementation also causes a decrease in proinflammatory cytokine secretion and downregulates apoptosis pathways during *Salmonella* infection [33]. Similarly, proteomic signatures of the spleen revealed that the actions of SDP are anti-inflammatory and anti-apoptotic and predicted to inhibit proinflammatory response through the inhibition of NF-κB. Protein phosphorylation such as FES, GSK3A, PKN3, BECN1, SMG1, and CASK were enriched with SDP treatment in the presence of *Salmonella*. Overall, proteins that decreased were associated with positive regulation of I-kappaß kinase/NF- kappaß signaling and positive regulation of apoptosis process while proteins that increased were associated with integral components of endoplasmic reticulum membrane and necroptosis pathway. This suggests that SDP plays a role in regulating immune response in the intestine via protein phosphorylation mechanism, thereby enhancing intestinal barrier integrity, gut microflora balance, and overall livestock wellbeing (**Table 3**) [34].

Furthermore, plant extracts such as onion peel extracts, green tea, onion peel, and garlic contain numerous bioactive compounds, including polyphenols, shogaols, quercetin, terpenes, gingerols, and phytosterols. These compounds have antioxidants,

Activities that occur during Salmonella infection with SDP treatment	Decrease in protein abundance	Increase in protein abundance
NF-kappaB signaling	RELA, TRADD, CANT1, TFG, and RIPK2	
Apoptosis pathway	TRADD, CTSL, RELA	
Protein phosphorylation		FES, GSK3A, PKN3, BECN1, SMG1, CASK

Table 3.
Increase and decrease in abundance of proteins during Salmonella *infection with SDP treatment.*

immunomodulatory, and antibacterial properties, and as a result, they influence the metabolism of energy, cell membrane activities, and nucleic acid production [35]. For instance, thymol, eugenol, and carvacrol, extracted from oregano and clove, disrupt bacterial cell walls, resulting in the leaking of intracellular contents and subsequent cell death [36]. Also, plant extracts such as *Curcuma* and *Scullaria* plant have been reported to decreased inflammation in chickens infected with *Salmonella* [37]. Particularly, the action of these plants as it relates to *Salmonella* infection mitigation have been attributed to their ability to modulate immune signaling pathways by attenuating the overexpression of proinflammatory cytokines such as IL-1β, IL-6, and TNF-α, frequently via the inhibition of NF-κB and MAPK pathways [37, 38]. Notably, the expression of inflammatory cytokines such as IL6, IL8L2, CASP6 and IRF7 were downregulated with the addition of Intebio (a commercial phytobiotic product) in the presence of *Salmonella Gallinarium* infection [38]. Overall, these bioactive compounds demonstrate direct bactericidal or bacteriostatic effects on Salmonella spp. by targeting the bacterial membrane, disrupting ATP synthesis, and interfering with DNA replication [38]. The anti-inflammatory property is crucial during Salmonella infection, since increased cytokine production may lead to intestinal tissue damage and impairment of epithelial barrier function and lowered intestinal absorption and livestock growth. Thus, certain phytochemicals, like quercetin and curcumin, augment the antioxidant defense system by upregulating glutathione peroxidase (GPx), superoxide dismutase (SOD), and catalase, therefore diminishing oxidative stress in intestinal tissues [39]. In protecting intestinal barrier integrity against intestinal colonization by *Salmonella* in the jejunum tissues and crypts, Eugenol has been used to not only downregulate proinflammatory cytokines IL-1β, IL-6, and TNF-α and inhibited the activation of JAK2/STAT3 signaling pathway [40]. Similarly, phytobiotics have been used to regulate and mitigate the immune system and inflammatory damage, respectively [41].

4. Conclusion

Overall, the mechanism of action of *Salmonella* involves the recruitment of cytokines via the NF-κB pathway and autophagy of infected cells, leading to a diversion of energy from developmental and physiological processes. This action results in anemia, malabsorption, and a physical decrease in growth rate and animal performance. In mitigating *Salmonella* action, BMD prevents the secretion of proinflammatory cytokines and ensures the selective removal of the abnormally folded protein, thereby maintaining a balance in the system. Similarly, SDP and plant extracts containing

DOI: http://dx.doi.org/10.5772/intechopen.1011658

bioactive compounds modulate intestinal microflora, improve antioxidant capacity, and decrease proinflammatory cytokine secretion leading to an increase in livestock performance.

Conflict of interest

The authors declare no conflict of interest.

Author details

Adedeji O. Adetunji[1*], Heidi Price[1], Henrietta Owusu[1], Emmanuel Asiamah[1] and Olumuyiwa Olarotimi[2]

1 Department of Agriculture, University of Arkansas at Pine Bluff, Pine Bluff, AR, USA

2 Department of Animal Science, Faculty of Agriculture, Adekunle Ajasin University, Akungba-Akoko, Ondo State, Nigeria

*Address all correspondence to: adetunjia@uapb.edu

References

[1] Barrow PA, Freitas Neto OC. Salmonella infections in pigs: A review. Brazilian Journal of Veterinary Research and Animal Science. 2011;**48**(2):89-98

[2] Boyen F, Haesebrouck F, Maes D, Van Immerseel F, Ducatelle R, Pasmans F. Non-typhoidal Salmonella infections in pigs: A closer look at epidemiology, pathogenesis and control. Veterinary Microbiology. 2008;**130**(1-2):1-19

[3] Hansen-Wester I, Hensel M. Salmonella pathogenicity islands encoding type III secretion systems. Microbes and Infection. 2001;**3**(7):549-559

[4] Adetunji A, Casey T, Franco J, Shah D, Fasina Y. Proteomic analysis of the effect of Salmonella challenge on broiler chicken. Molecules. 2022;**27**(21):7277. DOI: 10.3390/molecules27217277

[5] Galán JE. Salmonella interactions with host cells: Type III secretion at work. Annual Review of Cell and Developmental Biology. 2001;**17**:53-86

[6] Hensel M. Salmonella pathogenicity island 2. Molecular Microbiology. 2000;**36**(5):1015-1023

[7] Haraga A, Ohlson MB, Miller SI. Salmonellae interplay with host cells. Nature Reviews. Microbiology. 2008;**6**(1):53-66

[8] Santos RL, Zhang S, Tsolis RM, Kingsley RA, Adams LG, Bäumler AJ. Animal models of *Salmonella* infections: Enteritis versus typhoid fever. Microbes and Infection. 2001;**3**(14-15):1335-1344

[9] Tsolis RM, Xavier MN, Santos RL, Bäumler AJ. How to become a top model: Impact of animal experimentation on human *Salmonella* disease research. Infection and Immunity. 2011;**79**(5):1806-1814

[10] Hutchings MI, Truman AW, Wilkinson B. Antibiotics: Past, present and future. Current Opinion in Microbiology. 2019;**51**:72-80. DOI: 10.1016/j.mib.2019.10.008

[11] Adetunji AO, Price J, Owusu H, Adewale EF, Adesina PA, Saliu TP, et al. Mechanisms by which phytogenic extracts enhance livestock reproductive health: Current insights and future directions. Frontiers in Veterinary Science. 2025;**12**:1568577. DOI: 10.3389/fvets.2025.1568577

[12] Blue CEC, Jababu Y, Ibrahim SA, et al. Spray-dried plasma promotes broiler chick growth by enhancing immune surveillance. Animals (Basel). 2023;**13**(9):1436. DOI: 10.3390/ani13091436

[13] Fasina YO, Obanla TO, Ferket PR, Shah DH. Comparative efficacy of spray-dried plasma and bacitracin methylene disalicylate in reducing cecal colonization by *Salmonella enteritidis* in broiler chickens. Poultry Science. 2021;**100**:101134. DOI: 10.1016/j.psj.2020.101134

[14] Cosby DE, Cox NA, Harrison MA, Wilson JL, Buhr RJ, Fedora-Cray PJ. Salmonella and antimicrobial resistance in broilers: A review. Poultry Science. 2015;**94**(10):2446-2454. DOI: 10.3382/ps/pev190

[15] Davies RH, Wray C. Distribution of *Salmonella* contamination in ten animal feed mills. Veterinary Microbiology. 1997;**51**(1-2):159-169

[16] Lamichhane B, Mawad AMM, Saleh M, Kelley WG, Harrington PJ 2nd,

Lovestad CW, et al. Salmonellosis: An overview of epidemiology, pathogenesis, and innovative approaches to mitigate the antimicrobial resistant infections. Antibiotics (Basel). 2024;**13**(1):76. DOI: 10.3390/antibiotics13010076

[17] Belloy L, Decrausaz L, Boujon P, Hächler H, Waldvogel AS. Diagnosis by culture and PCR of *Salmonella abortusovis* infection under clinical conditions in aborting sheep in Switzerland. Veterinary Microbiology. 2009;**138**(3-4):373-377

[18] Uzzau S, Marogna G, Leori GS, Curtiss R, Schianchi G, Stocker BAD, et al. Virulence attenuation and live vaccine potential of aroA, crp, cdt, cya, and plasmid-cured mutants of *Salmonella enterica* serovar abortusovis in mice and sheep. Infection and Immunity. 2005;**73**(7):4302-4308. DOI: 10.1128/iai.73.7.4302-4308.2005

[19] Bonardi S. Salmonella in the pork production chain and its impact on human health in the European Union. Epidemiology and Infection. 2017;**145**(8):1513-1526. DOI: 10.1017/S095026881700036X

[20] Soliani L, Rugna G, Prosperi A, Chiapponi C, Luppi A. Salmonella infection in pigs: Disease, prevalence, and a link between swine and human health. Pathogens. 2023;**12**(10):1267. DOI: 10.3390/pathogens12101267

[21] Billah MM, Rahman MS. Salmonella in the environment: A review on ecology, antimicrobial resistance, seafood contaminations, and human health implications. Journal of Hazardous Materials Advances. 2024;**13**:100407. DOI: 10.1016/j.hazadv.2024.100407

[22] Evangelopoulou G, Kritas S, Govaris A, Burriel AR. Pork meat as a potential source of *Salmonella enterica* subsp. *arizonae* infection in humans. Journal of Clinical Microbiology. 2014;**52**(3):741-744. DOI: 10.1128/JCM.02933-13

[23] Holschbach CL, Peek SF. Salmonella in dairy cattle. The Veterinary Clinics of North America. Food Animal Practice. 2018;**34**(1):133-154. Available from: https://pmc.ncbi.nlm.nih.gov/articles/PMC7135009/

[24] Velasquez-Munoz A, Castro-Vargas R, Cullens-Nobis FM, Mani R, Abuelo A. Review: *Salmonella Dublin* in dairy cattle. Frontiers in Veterinary Science. 2024;**10**:1331767. DOI: 10.3389/fvets.2023.1331767

[25] Troeger H, Loddenkemper C, Schneider T, et al. Structural and functional changes of the duodenum in human norovirus infection. Gut. 2009;**58**:1070-1077

[26] Broberg S, Sahlin K. Adenine nucleotide degradation in human skeletal muscle during prolonged exercise. Journal of Applied Physiology. 1989;**67**(1):116-122

[27] Adetunji A, Casey T, Aryal UK, Ogundare T, Franco J, Fasina Y. Bacitracin methylene disalicylate (BMD) treatment affects spleen proteome in broiler chicks infected with *Salmonella enteritidis*. Antibiotics (Basel). 2024;**13**(5):414. DOI: 10.3390/antibiotics13050414

[28] Lecker SH, Goldberg AL, Mitch WE. Protein degradation by the ubiquitin-proteasome pathway in normal and disease states. Journal of the American Society of Nephrology. 2006;**17**(7):1807-1819

[29] Pérez-Bosque A, Miró L, Amat C, Polo J, Moretó M. The anti-inflammatory effect of spray-dried plasma is mediated by a reduction in mucosal lymphocyte

activation and infiltration in a mouse model of intestinal inflammation. Nutrients. 2016;**8**(10):657. DOI: 10.3390/nu8100657

[30] Zhang Y, Chen DW, Yu B, He J, Yu J, Mao XB, et al. Spray-dried chicken plasma improves intestinal digestive function and regulates intestinal selected microflora in weaning piglets. Journal of Animal Science. 2015;**93**(6):2967-2976. DOI: 10.2527/jas.2014-8820

[31] Pont GCD, Lee A, Bortoluzzi C, Farnell Y, Gougoulias C, Kogut M. Novel model for chronic intestinal inflammation in chickens: (2) immunologic mechanism behind the inflammatory response. Developmental and Comparative Immunology. 2022;**138**:104524. DOI: 10.1016/j.dci.2022.104524

[32] Campbell JM, Crenshaw JD, González-Esquerra R, Polo J. Impact of spray-dried plasma on intestinal health and broiler performance. Microorganisms. 2019;7(8):219. DOI: 10.3390/microorganisms7080219

[33] Obanla TO, Khan MM, Adetunji AO, Ajuwon KM, Fahrenholz AC, Iwuozo OC, et al. Characterization of spray-dried plasma-induced immune response in *Salmonella*-challenged broiler chicks. Poultry Science. 2024;**103**(11):104077. DOI: 10.1016/j.psj.2024.104077

[34] Ogundare TE, Casey TM, Aryal UK, Fasina YO. Spleen proteome profile reveals immune responses induced by dietary spray-dried plasma against *Salmonella enteritidis* infection in broiler chicks. Poultry Science. 2025;**104**(5):103330. DOI: 10.1016/j.psj.2024.103330

[35] Zhang L, Ravipati AS, Koyyalamudi SR, Jeong SC, Reddy N, Smith PT, et al. Antioxidant and anti-inflammatory activities of selected medicinal plants containing phenolic and flavonoid compounds. Journal of Agricultural and Food Chemistry. 2011;**59**(23):12361-12367. DOI: 10.1021/jf202511k

[36] Kalemba D, Kunicka A. Antibacterial and antifungal properties of essential oils. Current Medicinal Chemistry. 2003;**10**(10):813-829. DOI: 10.2174/0929867033457719

[37] Varmuzova K, Matulova ME, Gerzova L, Cejkova D, Gardan-Salmon D, Panhéleux M, et al. Curcuma and Scutellaria plant extracts protect chickens against inflammation and Salmonella enteritidis infection. Poultry Science. 2015;**94**(9):2049-2058. DOI: 10.3382/ps/pev190

[38] Anand P, Kunnumakkara AB, Newman RA, Aggarwal BB. Bioavailability of curcumin: Problems and promises. Molecular Pharmaceutics. 2007;**4**(6):807-818. DOI: 10.1021/mp700113r

[39] Lv Y, Zeng N, Feng Y, Zhang S, Zhou X, Gao C. Eugenol accelerates intestinal stem cell regeneration to protect the intestinal barrier integrity through inhibiting JAK2/STAT3 signaling pathway in *Salmonella enteritidis*-challenged broiler chicks. Journal of Animal Science and Biotechnology. 2025;**16**(1):40. DOI: 10.1186/s40104-025-01168-y

[40] Angane M, Swift S, Huang K, Perera J, Chen X, Butts CA, et al. Synergistic antimicrobial interaction of plant essential oils and extracts against foodborne pathogens. Food Science & Nutrition. 2024;**12**:1189-1206. DOI: 10.1002/fsn3.3834

[41] Shaji S, Selvaraj RK, Shanmugasundaram R. Salmonella infection in poultry: A review on the pathogen and control strategies. Microorganisms. 2023;**11**(11):2814. DOI: 10.3390/microorganisms11112814

Section 3

Adverse Reactions and Alternative Treatments

Chapter 7

Skin Adverse Reactions of *Salmonella* Infections

Melis Gönülal

Abstract

Salmonella species primarily cause infections in the gastrointestinal system, namely diarrhea, abdominal cramps and pain, nausea, vomiting, fever, and chills. Extra-intestinal focal infections include septic arthritis, osteomyelitis, cholangitis, aortitis, endocarditis, pneumonia, urinary tract infection, and meningitis. Rarely they may also affect the skin. In the literature, cases with ulcerated nodules, erythema nodosum, cutaneous abscesses, leukocytoclastic vasculitis, carbuncle, scrotal ulceration, maculopapular rash, and Schoenlein-Henoch's disease have been reported, with these cutaneous findings attributed to *Salmonella* species. If patients with cutaneous infections and cutaneous rash apply to the outpatient clinics, clinicians should think *Salmonella* as a causative factor. Here, different cutaneous infections and rash are summarized in this topic.

Keywords: *Salmonella*, skin, advers reactions, cutaneous reactions, infection

1. Introduction

Within the vast bacterial family *Enterobacteriaceae*, the *Salmonella* genus showcases remarkable heterogeneity, boasting more than 2600 distinct serovars identified by their unique surface markers. These numerous variants are primarily classified into two significant categories: typhoidal *Salmonella* and non-typhoidal *Salmonella* (NTS). The former group, predominantly encompassing *Salmonella Typhi* along with *Salmonella Paratyphi* A, B, and C, has evolved to specifically target human hosts, instigating the severe conditions known as typhoid and paratyphoid fevers. Such invasive illnesses are typically marked by persistent fever and widespread bodily indicators, often culminating in serious health issues if proper medical intervention is not administered. In contrast, NTS serovars, notably *Salmonella Enteritidis* and *Salmonella Typhimurium*, are more frequently implicated in bouts of acute stomach flu. A key challenge in managing NTS is their capacity to colonize diverse animal species, which then act as natural reservoirs, complicating efforts to limit human exposure [1, 2].

While *Salmonella* infections are primarily known for their impact on the gastrointestinal tract, leading to conditions ranging from self-limiting gastroenteritis to severe typhoid fever, they can also give rise to a variety of cutaneous manifestations. These skin changes, though less common than enteric symptoms, can provide important diagnostic clues, especially in cases of disseminated or systemic infection, and may occasionally be the presenting sign. Understanding the spectrum of these dermatological presentations is crucial for clinicians, as they can sometimes herald more serious underlying disease [3, 4].

1.1 The "rose spots"of typhoid fever

The most classic and recognized cutaneous manifestation associated with *Salmonella* infection is the "rose spot" rash seen in typhoid fever, caused by *Salmonella Typhi* (and occasionally *Salmonella Paratyphi*). These are faint, salmon-colored, macular or maculopapular lesions, typically 2–4 mm in diameter, that blanch on pressure. They appear in crops, most commonly on the trunk and upper abdomen, but can also be found on the chest or back. The rash usually emerges during the second week of illness, often coinciding with the peak of the fever, and may last for only a few days. Histologically, rose spots are characterized by localized inflammation of the dermis, perivascular infiltration of mononuclear cells, and the presence of *Salmonella* bacteria within the lesions. While historically considered a hallmark sign, rose spots are not always present and can be subtle, sometimes requiring careful examination, especially in individuals with darker skin tones where they may be less apparent. Their transient nature and often sparse distribution mean they can easily be missed. Despite their classic description, the absence of rose spots does not rule out a diagnosis of typhoid fever [5].

1.2 NTS and skin involvement

Beyond typhoid fever, NTS infections, which are far more prevalent globally, can also lead to dermatological issues, although these are generally less specific and occur predominantly in patients with bacteremia or those who are immunocompromised. Unlike the classic rose spots of typhoid, NTS-associated skin lesions are highly variable and often indicative of systemic dissemination of the bacteria. One common presentation in NTS bacteremia is a macular or maculopapular rash, which may be widespread and can sometimes resemble viral exanthems. These rashes are typically non-specific and are thought to result from the systemic inflammatory response to the circulating bacteria. In some severe cases, pustular lesions, nodules, or even abscesses may develop, particularly in individuals with compromised immune systems (e.g., HIV/AIDS patients, transplant recipients, or those on immunosuppressive therapy). These more severe skin lesions usually represent focal metastatic infection, where *Salmonella* bacteria have seeded the skin directly from the bloodstream. Such lesions can be tender, erythematous, and may lead to necrosis if left untreated. Furthermore, NTS can be a rare cause of cellulitis, a bacterial skin infection characterized by redness, swelling, and warmth, often occurring at sites of preexisting skin trauma or lesions. Ecthyma gangrenosum-like lesions, typically seen in *Pseudomonas aeruginosa* infections, have also been rarely reported in severe NTS bacteremia, particularly in severely immunocompromised individuals. These are necrotic ulcers with a distinctive violaceous border [6, 7].

1.3 Reactive arthropathy and other immune-mediated skin reactions

Beyond direct bacterial presence in the skin, *Salmonella* infections, particularly NTS, are well-known triggers for reactive arthropathy (formerly Reiter's syndrome). This sterile inflammatory arthritis typically develops days to weeks after the acute gastrointestinal infection. While primarily affecting joints, reactive arthritis can also be accompanied by specific mucocutaneous manifestations. These include keratoderma blennorrhagicum, which are psoriasiform lesions on the palms and soles that can resemble pustular psoriasis, and circinate balanitis, a rash on the glans penis. Oral ulcers may also be present. These skin conditions are not due to the direct presence of the bacteria but are immune-mediated phenomena, a delayed hypersensitivity reaction to the *Salmonella* antigens. The skin involvement in reactive arthropathy can be persistent and challenging to manage. In rare instances, *Salmonella* infection has also been implicated in triggering other immune-mediated skin conditions, such as erythema nodosum, characterized by tender, red nodules, typically on the shins, reflecting inflammation of subcutaneous fat. This is also considered a reactive process rather than direct infection [8–10].

1.4 Diagnostic challenges and clinical significance

The varied and often non-specific nature of *Salmonella*-associated skin lesions presents diagnostic challenges. A high index of suspicion is required, especially in the context of persistent fever, gastrointestinal symptoms, or immunocompromise. When skin lesions are observed, particularly atypical or persistent ones, biopsy of the lesion for histopathological examination and bacterial culture can be invaluable for confirming *Salmonella* involvement and guiding appropriate antibiotic therapy. For suspected reactive phenomena, clinical correlation with recent *Salmonella* infection and the presence of associated symptoms (e.g., arthritis) is key [3, 4].

To summarize, while not the most common feature, skin manifestations of *Salmonella* infections range from the classical rose spots of typhoid fever to various non-specific rashes, nodules, or even severe necrotic lesions in NTS bacteremia. Furthermore, *Salmonella* can trigger immune-mediated dermatological conditions such as keratoderma blennorrhagicum in reactive arthropathy. Recognizing these diverse skin findings is important for timely diagnosis, especially in complicated or systemic *Salmonella* infections, potentially prompting earlier and more effective management and improving patient outcomes [1–4].

We will investigate this topic based on current literature information.

2. Literature review

A case study documented the presentation of a 35-year-old female patient to a dermatology clinic, reporting a moderately tender, ulcerated nodule on the outer aspect of her right lower limb that had developed over several months. This lesion emerged weeks following her travel through Bangladesh. Initial diagnostic workup, including standard laboratory assays and radiographs of both the affected limb and chest, yielded no abnormalities. Histopathological examination similarly provided no definitive findings. However, repeated bacteriological cultures of samples obtained from the cutaneous ulcer ultimately identified *Salmonella typhi* as the etiological agent. The patient received a 15-day course of oral ciprofloxacin at 500 mg twice daily, resulting in complete resolution of the nodule, though residual hyperpigmentation and scarring were noted [11].

Huckstep's research, which examined a cohort of 240 adult individuals diagnosed with typhoid fever, revealed that between 2 and 9% of these patients developed subcutaneous abscesses attributed to *Salmonella typhi*. Notably, none of these specific cases presented with concurrent ulceration [12].

A case report detailed the experience of a two-year-old girl who presented with a non-specific fever for 2 weeks. Subsequently, she developed elevated, pigmented skin lesions over both greater trochanters. Within days, these painful lesions spontaneously ruptured, releasing a thick, creamy discharge. Examination revealed two ulcers: one measuring approximately 3–4 cm in diameter and 0.5 cm deep above each femoral trochanter, and another on the left side featuring a central piece of necrotic skin. All lesions exhibited surrounding induration. Bacteriological analysis of swabs taken from both ulcers identified *S. dublin* as the causative agent. Treatment commenced with oral ampicillin 250 mg every 6 hours for 10 days, followed by a five-day course of chloramphenicol 0.5 g. The ulcers achieved complete resolution within 1 month [13].

Various *Salmonella* species have been implicated in the development of erythema nodosum, with a total of 28 cases documented in the existing literature to date. The reported causative agents in these instances include diverse serotypes such as *Salmonella enteritidis*, *Salmonella enterica* serotype Poona, and *Salmonella typhimurium*. Furthermore, specific clinical presentations like *Salmonella enteritidis* enteritis, *Salmonella typhimurium* enteritis, *Salmonella enteritidis* gastroenteritis, *Salmonella enteritidis* enterocolitis, and general *Salmonella* gastroenteritis have been identified as preceding events [14–19]. **Table 1** provides details on some of these individual case reports.

Beyond other skin manifestations, *Salmonella* species are also capable of causing cutaneous abscesses. To date, eight case reports detailing such occurrences have been documented in medical literature. A variety of *Salmonella* serotypes, including *Salmonella Enterica* subsp., *Salmonella enterica* serotype Choleraesuis, *Salmonella* group D, *Salmonella typhi*, *Salmonella enteritidis*, *Salmonella adelaide*, and *Salmonella typhimurium*, have been identified in these skin abscesses [20].

A notable instance is presented in the case report by Chiao et al. [21], involving a 30-year-old male with diabetes mellitus who developed a painful nodule on his

***Salmonella* type (reference)**	**Gender/age**	**Locations of the lesions**	**Laboratory and scanning findings**	**Treatment**
Salmonella enteritidis [15]	Female/26	The left lower limb	Lower limb ultrasonography; subcutaneous edema with no loculated fluid collection	Oral ciprofloxacin (500 mg) every 12 h
Salmonella enteritidis [16]	Male/8	Both shins	Normal	Ampicillin 150 mg/kg/day divided in equal doses four times/day for 10 days
Salmonella enterica Serotype Poona [17]	Female/23	both shins	Normal	Ciprofloxacin 400 mg every 12 h for 9 days.
Salmonella gastroenteritis [18]	Female/21	Both legs	Normal	Salicylates
Salmonella [19]	?/7	Both legs	White blood cell, neutrophil, platelets, C-reactive protein are high	Symptomatic treatment of pain and antibiotics

Table 1.
Erythema nodosum lesions because of Salmonella.

anterior chest. He underwent sharp debridement and bacterial culture, which identified *Salmonella* group D, sensitive to ceftriaxone and ciprofloxacin. Intravenous ceftriaxone (2.0 g daily) was administered for 10 days, and surgical debridement of the wound was performed on the second hospital day. This procedure revealed a subcutaneous abscess, approximately 7 cm×4 cm, located beneath the ulcerative lesion. The patient was discharged a week post-surgery, with his antibiotic regimen transitioning to oral ciprofloxacin for an additional week.

Another reported case involved a 64-year-old woman who presented with a progressively enlarging mass in her lower back, accompanied by swelling and redness of the surrounding skin. Her laboratory tests indicated elevated white blood cell count, neutrophils, and C-reactive protein. Imaging studies, including a chest X-ray (CXR) and spinal MRI (T2-FRFSE, T1-FSE sequences), confirmed the presence of a spinal abscess [22]. These cases underscore the necessity of performing radiological imaging when *Salmonella*-induced abscesses are suspected, particularly for deeper or more extensive lesions.

The case report by Filiz et al. [23] describes a four-year-old girl with Interleukin-12 Receptor Beta-1 deficiency who was referred to a dermatology outpatient clinic due to recurring skin eruptions and lymphadenitis. Her presentation included edema and purpuric eruptions on her upper and lower extremities and abdomen. Laboratory findings showed elevated C-reactive protein and erythrocyte sedimentation rate. A skin biopsy revealed a dense inflammatory infiltrate rich in eosinophils, neutrophils, and fibrin within the upper dermis and dermal vessel walls, consistent with leukocytoclastic vasculitis. Serological testing for *Salmonella* agglutination was positive, and *S. enteritidis* was subsequently isolated from her blood culture. Following the initiation of ceftriaxone therapy, her lesions completely cleared within a few days.

Sulaiman et al. [24] documented five pediatric cases of cutaneous leukocytoclastic vasculitis, involving three girls and two boys aged 4–13 years. The isolated pathogens were *Salmonella* groups B, C, and D. All these patients had a history of recurrent *Salmonella* infections, presenting as enteritis, urinary tract infections, abscess formation, and sepsis. Management included appropriate antibiotic therapy for 2–4 weeks, with three patients requiring an additional 6 weeks of prophylactic treatment. For their vasculitis, three patients received naproxen, and two were given low-dose prednisone. Only one case of vasculitis was self-limiting.

Beyond other skin manifestations, *Salmonella* species can also cause carbuncles. One such instance involved a 55-year-old male with type 2 diabetes mellitus and hypertension who presented to the Emergency Department with a pus-discharging swelling (8 cm×6 cm) on the left side of his neck. The carbuncle was promptly incised and drained, and microbiological analysis of the pus culture identified *Salmonella*. In vitro susceptibility testing of the isolated *Salmonella* strain (CSE76F) was performed using the Vitek II system and E-test, with results interpreted according to Clinical and Laboratory Standards Institute (CLSI) guidelines. The patient began a 14-day course of intravenous ciprofloxacin at 400 mg every 12 hours. Following wound debridement, he was referred to plastic surgery for a skin graft [25].

Generalized maculopapular rashes can be a manifestation of *Salmonella* species infections. A case reported by Altamimi et al. [26] involved a four-year-old girl with IL12RB1 deficiency who presented with widespread urticarial macules and papules, accompanied by a few scattered purpuric lesions. This presentation followed a two-week history of recurrent fevers, a productive cough, and headache. Her chest, cardiovascular, and abdominal examinations were unremarkable. Blood cultures, taken upon admission, yielded *Salmonella* growth after 3 days. Treatment with meropenem was initiated, leading to an improvement of the rash, though post-inflammatory hyperpigmentation remained. She was eventually discharged on a regimen of linezolid, rifampicin, moxifloxacin, and fosfomycin.

Another case report documented a seven-year-old male presenting to the hospital with fever, a maculopapular rash, bloody and crusted lips, and exanthema overlying scutes. Stool analysis confirmed *Salmonella enteritidis*, and ceftriaxone treatment was initiated. By the fifth day of therapy, the patient's neurological, renal, and cardiorespiratory symptoms had markedly improved, and his maculopapular rash had also noticeably faded [27].

Between 1980 and 2008, Lee et al. [28] consulted or received referrals for 175 Taiwanese patients with primary immunodeficiency diseases at their institute, primarily for molecular diagnosis or treatment. Their investigation focused on identifying individuals with a defective IL-12/23-IFN-γ circuit. Among these patients, one case stood out: an individual with a missense IL12RB1 mutation (Arg211Pro) who experienced recurrent *Salmonella enteritidis* D sepsis and pneumatocele. The authors concluded that patients exhibiting an impaired IL-12/23-IFN-γ circuit might present with features resembling or overlapping with *Salmonella* pneumatocele.

Salmonella species can also cause scrotal ulcerations. A case report described a 16-year-old male who sought hospital admission for necrotic scrotal ulcerations that had developed over the preceding 3 weeks. This skin condition occurred alongside a systemic illness characterized by fever, diarrhea, weight loss, and a general decline in health. Testing confirmed a *Salmonella* infection. He began a three-week course of fluoroquinolone antibiotics, which led to complete healing by the end of that period [29].

Salmonella species can also be associated with Schoenlein-Henoch's disease (HSP). A case report detailed two young girls, aged 2 years and 8 months, and 13 months, respectively, who were hospitalized with diarrhea. Both presented with symmetrical, pompho-erythemato-hemorrhagic and petechial cutaneous lesions located on the extensor surfaces of their lower limbs and buttocks. *Salmonella* type C and D groups were identified in their stool and blood cultures. Both patients recovered after receiving appropriate antibiotic treatment [30].

In the work of Huang and DuPont [31], *Salmonella typhi* including its tendency for extra-intestinal seeding depends on several factors: the initial dose of ingested bacteria, the virulence of the *S. Typhi* strain, the host's immune response, prior exposure, and local protective elements but there is a problem that multidrug-resistant *S. Typhi* strains complicate treatment and contribute to a higher risk of severe complications and mortality, particularly in endemic regions. In this work especially rose spots had been mentioned as cutaneous reactions because of *Salmonella typhi*.

Malignancies, along with the chemotherapy or immunosuppressive treatments often associated with them, severely impair the body's ability to contain bacterial infections. This allows *Salmonella* to overcome local barriers and enter the bloodstream, subsequently seeding various organs, including the skin. While the precise nature of these skin lesions (e.g., abscesses, cellulitis, or less common reactive phenomena) might vary and require further investigation within the full text of such a review, the critical takeaway is the heightened susceptibility of these patients to systemic spread that can manifest cutaneously. Therefore, for clinicians managing patients with disseminated malignant diseases who present with any skin abnormalities, considering *Salmonella* as a potential cause, driven by its systemic dissemination, becomes an essential diagnostic consideration [32].

2.1 Salmonella vaccine

In the work of Baliban et al. [33] *Salmonella* vaccine-induced skin reactions typically involve the area where the injection was given. Common manifestations include erythema, edema, and tenderness or pain at the injection site. Such local reactions are a normal and anticipated part of the vaccination process, indicating an effective immune activation. While the review does not delve into detailed descriptions of specific skin lesion types beyond general reactogenicity, it acknowledges that these transient cutaneous responses are part of the safety profile evaluated during vaccine development. The focus remains on their mild and temporary nature, distinguishing them from more severe adverse events, and confirming that the vaccine candidates generally exhibit an acceptable safety profile regarding these common injection site effects.

Bellanti et al. [34] had been mentioned in their work about skin reactions because of *Salmonella* vaccine, these are especially local reactions such as pain, tenderness, redness erythema, and swelling. Some individuals might experience delayed hypersensitivity reactions, which can sometimes present as nodules at the injection site. These reactions, while less frequent than immediate local soreness or redness, are usually self-limiting. The general principles outlined in the article regarding vaccine safety and common reactions therefore suggest that *Salmonella* vaccines would similarly elicit these types of transient and usually minor dermatological responses at the injection site.

Adverse skin reactions caused by *Salmonella* vaccines are minor. The potential skin reactions can be considered insignificant when weighed against the benefits gained from *Salmonella* vaccines. Therefore, *Salmonella* vaccination is recommended, especially in endemic regions [34, 35].

3. Conclusion

When patients present in outpatient settings with a range of skin conditions, it is essential for healthcare providers to look beyond the obvious and consider less common, yet significant, underlying causes. While *Salmonella* infections are primarily associated with digestive tract issues, an increasing body of evidence, mainly from detailed case reports and series, underscores their capacity to manifest through various dermatological findings. This means that if individuals exhibit conditions such as ulcerated nodules, erythema nodosum, skin abscesses, leukocytoclastic vasculitis, carbuncles, scrotal ulcerations, maculopapular rashes, or Schoenlein-Henoch's disease, healthcare professionals should actively consider *Salmonella* as a potential contributing factor [1–3].

The most iconic skin sign of typhoid fever, caused by *Salmonella typhi*, is the "rose spot" rash. These subtle, temporary, salmon-hued spots on the torso, though sometimes overlooked, should immediately prompt investigation for systemic typhoid, especially in travelers returning from affected regions or during known outbreaks. However, *Salmonella*'s dermatological impact extends far beyond these faint lesions. For example, skin abscesses represent a direct bacterial invasion of the skin, often necessitating surgical drainage in addition to antibiotics. These can be particularly challenging in patients with weakened immune systems, where *Salmonella* serotypes might lead to deep, pus-filled pockets that could be missed if *Salmonella* is not suspected. Similarly, the documented occurrences of *Salmonella*-induced carbuncles—larger, interconnected pus collections—demonstrate the potential for severe localized skin infections demanding vigorous treatment [4–6].

Beyond direct bacterial presence, *Salmonella* infections are recognized triggers for several immune-mediated skin reactions. Erythema nodosum, characterized by tender, red lumps, typically on the shins, has been linked to *Salmonella* in numerous published cases. This condition arises from the body's immune response to the infection causing inflammation in the fatty layer beneath the skin, rather than direct bacterial presence. Similarly, leukocytoclastic vasculitis, an inflammation of small blood vessels in the skin leading to various purpuric or erythematous lesions, has been observed in conjunction with *Salmonella* infections, particularly in immunocompromised children. These immune-driven responses highlight the need for careful dermatological and infectious disease evaluation. The well-established link between *Salmonella* and reactive arthropathy (formerly Reiter's syndrome) also brings specific skin and mucous membrane manifestations like keratoderma blennorrhagicum (psoriasis-like lesions on palms and soles) and circinate balanitis. These instances underscore that *Salmonella*'s effect on the skin is not always direct but can be a complex interaction with the host's immune system [15–19].

The clinical implications of this broadened perspective are profound. Firstly, including *Salmonella* in the differential diagnosis for these varied skin conditions can lead to faster and more accurate diagnoses, especially when typical gastrointestinal symptoms are absent or minor. Delayed or incorrect diagnoses can prolong illness, lead to unnecessary tests, and potentially result in severe complications, particularly if the *Salmonella* infection is widespread or invasive. Secondly, recognizing these skin signs can guide the selection of appropriate antibiotic treatment. Given the global rise in *Salmonella* antimicrobial resistance, precise identification of the pathogen from skin lesions (through culture and susceptibility testing) is vital for targeted therapy, avoiding the misuse of broad-spectrum antibiotics [1, 8, 11].

Furthermore, being aware of these cutaneous indicators promotes a more thorough patient history, including recent travel, dietary habits, and immune status, which are crucial for assessing *Salmonella* risk. For instance, recurrent or persistent skin eruptions in an immunocompromised patient should always prompt a search for unusual opportunistic infections, including *Salmonella*. Diagnostic imaging, such as radiological scans, might also be necessary for deeper or more extensive abscesses [11].

While *Salmonella* species primarily target the digestive system, the wide array of associated skin manifestations, from direct infections to immune-mediated conditions, should not be underestimated. Clinicians examining patients with any of the previously mentioned skin conditions—be it ulcerated nodules, erythema nodosum, skin abscesses, leukocytoclastic vasculitis, carbuncles, scrotal ulcerations, maculopapular rashes, or Schoenlein-Henoch's disease—must expand their diagnostic thinking. Incorporating *Salmonella* into the differential diagnosis for these dermatological presentations is a vital step toward timely and precise diagnosis, enabling targeted treatment and ultimately enhancing patient outcomes against this adaptable bacterial pathogen.

DOI: http://dx.doi.org/10.5772/intechopen.1012201

Author details

Melis Gönülal[1,2]

1 Unit of Dermatology, İzmir Tepecik Training and Research Hospital, University of Health Sciences, İzmir, Turkey

2 Unit of Dermatology, İzmir Faculty of Medicine, University of Health Sciences, İzmir, Turkey

*Address all correspondence to: drmelis@gmail.com

References

[1] Balasubramanian R, Im J, Lee JS, Jeon HJ, Mogeni OD, Kim JH, et al. The global burden and epidemiology of invasive non-typhoidal *Salmonella* infections. Human Vaccines & Immunotherapeutics. 2019;**15**(6):1421-1426

[2] Meiring JE, Khanam F, Basnyat B, Charles RC, Crump JA, Debellut F, et al. Typhoid fever. Nature Reviews Disease Primers. 2023;**9**(1):71

[3] Parry CM, Hien TT, Dougan G, White NJ, Farrar JJ. Clinical manifestations of typhoid fever: A systematic review and meta-analysis. Transactions of the Royal Society of Tropical Medicine and Hygiene. 2005;**99**(12):991-1002

[4] Hohmann EL. Nontyphoidal *Salmonella* infections. Clinical Infectious Diseases. 2001;**32**(2):263-269

[5] Litwack KD, Hoke AW, Borchardt KA. Rose spots in typhoid fever. Archives of Dermatology. 1972;**105**(2):252-253. passim

[6] Von Roenn A, Serai J, Dondonan CR, Gemayel R, Brooks E. An intriguing case of non-typhoidal *Salmonella* presenting as bacteremia and bilateral cellulitis in a diabetic patient. Cureus. 2025;**17**(3):e80297

[7] Gordon MA, Banda HT, Gondwe M, Gordon SB, Walsh AL, Phiri A, et al. Non-typhoidal *Salmonella* (NTS) bacteraemia in Malawian adults: A severe, recrudescent, HIV-associated illness. Malawi Medical Journal. 2003;**15**(2):47-51

[8] Aitken-Saavedra J, Maturana-Ramirez A, Fernández Moraga J, Doro Dias V, Galdino-Santos L, Pineda Flores D. Reactive arthritis: Images. Dermatology Online Journal. 2021;**27**:7

[9] Ajene AN, Fischer Walker CL, Black RE. Enteric pathogens and reactive arthritis: A systematic review of *Campylobacter*, *Salmonella* and *Shigella*-associated reactive arthritis. Journal of Health, Population, and Nutrition. 2013;**31**(3):299-307

[10] Catinean A, Neag MA, Mitre AO, Bocsan CI, Buzoianu AD. Microbiota and immune-mediated skin diseases-an overview. Microorganisms. 2019;**7**(9):279

[11] Marzano AV, Mercogliano M, Borghi A, Facchetti M, Caputo R. Cutaneous infection caused by *Salmonella typhi*. Journal of the European Academy of Dermatology and Venereology. 2003;**17**(5):575-577

[12] Huckstep RL. Typhoid Fever and Other *Salmonella* Infections. Edinburgh and London: E. & S. Livingstone Ltd.; 1962. pp. 350

[13] Carswell W, Magrath IT. Skin ulceration caused by *Salmonella dublin*. British Medical Journal. 1973;**1**:331-332

[14] Castilla Cortázar A, Pastor Rodríguez A, Montejo Baranda M, Aguirre Errasti C. Salmonella gastroenteritis and erythema nodosum. Canadian Medical Association Journal. 15 Jul 1985;**133**(2):120

[15] Hassan A, Alsaihati A, Shammari MA, Sharroufna M, Alaithan H, Aljubran S. Erythema nodosum: A manifestation of *Salmonella* infection. Case Reports in Gastroenterology. 2019;**13**(3):456-461

[16] Mantadakis E, Arvanitidou V, Tsalkidis A, Thomaidis S, Chatzimichael A. Erythema nodosum associated with *Salmonella* enteritidis. Hippokratia. 2010;**14**(1):51-53

[17] Benwan KA, Mulla AA, Izumiya H, John AM. Erythema nodosum and bilateral breast abscesses due to *Salmonella enterica* serotype Poona. Journal of Clinical Microbiology. 2010;**48**(10):3786-3787

[18] Cortázar AC, Rodríguez AP, Baranda MM, Errasti CA. *Salmonella* gastroenteritis and erythema nodosum. Canadian Medical Association Journal. 1985;**133**(2):120

[19] Benhachem M, Hamami A, Elouali A, Babakhouya A, Rkain M. When *Salmonella* manifests through the skin: Erythema nodosum in a pediatric case. Cureus. 2024;**16**(6):e61594

[20] Sfeir M, Youssef P, Mokhbat JE. *Salmonella typhi* sternal wound infection. American Journal of Infection Control. Dec 2013;**41**(12):e123-4

[21] Chiao HY, Wang CY, Wang CH. Salmonella Abscess of the Anterior Chest Wall in a Patient With Type 2 Diabetes and Poor Glycemic Control: A Case Report. Ostomy Wound Manage. 2016;**62**(3):46-9

[22] Zaalishvili Z, Didbaridze T, Gogokhia N, Asanidze B, Akhmeteli L, Saginashvili L. *Salmonella enteritidis* phlegmon in an elderly female: A case report. Cureus. 2022;**14**(8):e27545

[23] Filiz S, Uygun DFK, Verhard EM, van Dissel JT, Uygun V, Bassorgun C. Cutaneous leukocytoclastic vasculitis due to *Salmonella enteritidis* in a child with interleukin-12 receptor beta-1 deficiency. Pediatric Dermatology. 2014;**31**(2):236-240

[24] Al-Mayouf SM, Bahabri S, Majeed M. Cutaneous leukocytoclastic vasculitis associated with mycobacterial and *Salmonella* infection. Clinical Rheumatology. 2007;**26**(9):1563-1564

[25] Alfouzan W, Bulach D, Izumiya H, AlBassam K, Sheikh S, Alrubai'aan N, et al. Carbuncle due to *Salmonella Enteritidis*: A novel presentation. Gut Pathogens. 2017;**11**(9):51

[26] Altamimi AM, Qadoumi TA, Alajroush W, Alzomia MA, Aljarbou O. The hidden cause of maculopapular rash in interleukin-12 deficiency. Cureus. 2022;**14**(1):e21415

[27] Wiegand G, Rauch R, Hermann M, Apitz C, Hofbeck M, Heininger U. *Salmonella enteritidis* infection presenting with septic shock, renal failure and cutaneous manifestations. Klinische Pädiatrie. 2009;**221**(1): 41-43

[28] Lee WI, Huang JL, Lin TY, Hsueh C, Wong AM, Hsieh MY, et al. Chinese patients with defective IL-12/23-interferon-gamma circuit in Taiwan: Partial dominant interferon-gamma receptor 1 mutation presenting as cutaneous granuloma and IL-12 receptor beta1 mutation as pneumatocele. Journal of Clinical Immunology. 2009;**29**(2):238-245

[29] Amraoui ME, Hjira N. A rare and atypical cause of scrotal ulcerations. The Pan African Medical Journal. 2018;**30**(29):87

[30] Zucchini A, Manfredi R. Schoenlein-Henoch syndrome and *Salmonella* infection: A new association? Minerva Pediatrica. 1992;**44**(11):559-563

[31] Huang DB, DuPont HL. Problem pathogens: Extra-intestinal complications of *Salmonella enterica*

serotype typhi infection. The Lancet Infectious Diseases. 2005;**5**(6):341-348

[32] Han T, Sokal JE, Neter E. Salmonellosis in disseminated malignant diseases: A seven-year review (1959-1965). The New England Journal of Medicine. 1967;**276**(19):1045-1052

[33] Baliban SM, Lu YJ, Malley R. Overview of the nontyphoidal and paratyphoidal *Salmonella* vaccine pipeline: Current status and future prospects. Clinical Infectious Diseases. 2020;**71**(Suppl. 2):S151-S154

[34] Bellanti JA, Fishman HJ, Wientzen RL. Adverse reactions to vaccines. Immunology and Allergy Clinics of North America. 1987;**7**(3):423-445

[35] Desin TS, Köster W, Potter AA. *Salmonella* vaccines in poultry: past, present and future. Expert Review of Vaccines. 2013;**12**(1):87-96

Chapter 8

Salmonellosis Infections and Treatment Proposals

Obou Constantin Okou and Margery Claude-Charlène Keke

Abstract

Enterobacteriaceae are among the most widespread bacteria in the world, and the most frequently encountered in clinical consultations. Unfortunately, these disease-causing germs are now increasingly resistant to the standard antibiotics generally used. In order to propose probable therapeutic alternatives, this study focused on evaluating the antibacterial activity of *Solanum torvum* fruit (a food plant) on around thirty strains of enterobacteria such as *Escherichia coli*, *Salmonella sp*, *Shigella sp*, *Citrobacter koseri*, *Enterobacter cloacae*, *Klebsiella pneumoniae*, *Proteus mirabilis*, and *Citrobacter freundii*. Among these strains of enterobacteria were nine strains of *Salmonella sp*. To do this, 70% hydroethanolic and 100% ethanolic extracts were prepared from the fruits of *Solanum torvum* and then tested on them. All strains of *Salmonella sp.* were isolated from various biological samples (stool and/or urine) from patients. Qualitative and quantitative analyses revealed the presence of several phytocompounds such as polyphenols, tannins, coumarins, saponosides, and so on in the 70% hydroethanolic and 100% ethanolic extracts. Finally, the antioxidant activity of both extracts showed that they were capable of inhibiting free radicals. The results revealed that these various extracts have antibacterial activity with a bactericidal effect on these strains. These extracts could therefore be used to produce phytomedicines to combat *Salmonella* infections.

Keywords: Salmonellosis, medicinal plants, antibacterial, antioxidant activities, phytocompounds

1. Introduction

Enterobacteriaceae are Gram-negative bacilli comprising 40 genera and over 130 species. They are found in humans, animals, and the environment [1, 2]. They are present in the digestive systems of humans and animals [3, 4]. They are a constant cause of urinary tract, pulmonary, and intra-abdominal infections; bacteremia; and meningitis and are encountered both in the community and in hospitals. *Escherichia*, *Salmonella*, *Shigella*, *Yersinia*, *Klebsiella*, *Enterobacter*, *Serratia*, *Morganella*, *Proteus*, *Providencia*, and *Citrobacter* are the most common pathogens [1, 5].

Over the last few decades, the overuse and/or inappropriate use of antibiotics has led to therapeutic failures with these bacteria. In fact, they can produce extended-spectrum β-lactamases (ESBLs) that can inhibit beta-lactam antibiotics. These enzymes can render antibiotics such as aminoglycosides and fluoroquinolones ineffective. This situation represents a real public health problem [6, 7]. Indeed, ESBL infections can increase overall patient morbidity and mortality. Consequently, around 700,000 deaths worldwide are due to antimicrobial resistance [4, 5, 8]. Therapeutic failures are prompting research teams to turn their attention to traditional African pharmacopoeia. Indeed, the WHO confirms that in Africa, 80% of the population relies on traditional medicine and pharmacopoeia to deal with health problems [9]. According to reference [10], the constant reinforcement of antimicrobial compounds through the discovery of new molecules keeps us one step ahead of the risk of therapeutic impasses. However, modern medicine is characterized by a crying lack of new treatments. What's more, antibiotics, regarded as the almost universal solution to serious infections, are increasingly showing their limitations [11, 12]. In this context, traditional medicine can provide a solution to these problems, as it is of prime importance in the health care of populations. As reference studies [13–15] have shown, medicinal plants have always been used for their cosmetic, chemical, dietetic, pharmaceutical, agri-food, and industrial properties. In particular, the work of reference studies [16–20] has shown that medicinal plants contain various biologically active chemical principles capable of exerting antioxidant, anti-inflammatory, analgesic, antibacterial, and other activities. Similarly, according to reference [21], medicinal plants are part of the history of every continent. Specifically, they have been organized, documented, and passed down from generation to generation for centuries in China and India. In Africa, as reference [22] points out, there are almost 5000 medicinal species. This study was carried out with the aim of contributing to the scientific valorization of medicinal plants. It aims to evaluate the antibacterial activity of *Solanum torvum* fruits on a few strains of hospital-acquired salmonellosis.

2. General information on the *Salmonella* genus

It was first discovered by Theobald Smith (1859–1934) in 1885. It is a straight bacillus, about 3 μm long, aero-anaerobic and often motile, except for *S. gallinarum*. According to Le Minor and Kaufmann-White, it comprises two subspecies: *Salmonella enterica* and *Salmonella bongori*. *Salmonella enterica* comprises 6 subspecies (*indica, salamae, arizonae, diarizonae, houtenae,* and *enterica*) [23].

3. Pathogenicity of the genus *Salmonella*

Salmonellosis is a disease caused by the *Salmonella* genus. They remain a major health problem, especially in underdeveloped countries. *Salmonella* are responsible for both major and minor salmonellosis (non-typhoidal salmonellosis). Major salmonellosis is the cause of typhoid and paratyphoid fevers. Typhoid and paratyphoid fevers are strictly human pathologies caused by the serovars *S. Typhi*, *S. Paratyphi A*, *S. Paratyphi B*, and *S. Paratyphi C*, while minor salmonellosis is the cause of gastroenteritis due to food poisoning by serovars such as *S. typhimurium*, *S. enteritidis*, and *S. panama* [24, 25].

4. Antibiotics and definition

Antibiotics derive their name from two Greek words, anti: against, and bios: life. They are natural, semisynthetic, or synthetic substances capable of inhibiting or destroying the growth of bacteria without harming the body. They were discovered in

1929 by Alexander Flemming. He was the first to discover penicillin. This discovery made it possible to combat certain diseases and paved the way for the discovery of several other molecules between 1940 and 2005. Antibiotics are therefore a large group of drugs composed of several families depending on their mode of action on bacteria and their chemical structures [7, 10, 26, 27].

5. Some figures on bacterial resistance

Bacterial resistance to antibiotics is becoming increasingly significant and is characterized by the emergence of new forms of resistance [28, 29]. This, according to reference [30], represents one of the major health challenges of the twenty-first century. The Organization for Economic Cooperation and Development (OECD) estimates that 2.4 million people in Europe, North America, and Australia will die from multidrug-resistant bacterial infections (MRB) over the next 30 years [31, 32]. In Europe, antibiotic-resistant bacteria cause 400,000 infections per year, with at least 25,000 deaths annually [33, 34]. In Africa, this phenomenon of resistance is poorly assessed. Nonetheless, studies report that the African continent is not immune to this phenomenon [34, 35]. Nevertheless, reference studies [36, 37] predict that by 2050, approximately 4.1 million people living in Africa will lose their lives due to MRB infections.

6. General information on the therapeutic use of *Solanum torvum*

In Dominica, the young leaves of *Solanum torvum* are used in combination with the leafy stem of *Bidens pilosa* to treat dysuria, and its flowers are used to treat abdominal pain in infants in the form of an infusion. In Guadeloupe, the roots macerated in water are used to treat renal colic [38]. In Cameroon, a decoction of the fruit is used to treat female infertility [39], and the bark, fruit, and leaves are used to treat poisoning, gastric problems, female infertility, and pneumonia [40]. In Central America, India, and Gabon, the leaves are used to treat cuts, wounds, and diabetes [41]. In Ghana, the leaves are used to treat wounds and boils [42], and in southern Nigeria, they are used to treat sickle cell anemia [43]. In southern Ivory Coast, a decoction of the leaves is used to treat anemia [44]. In Madagascar, a paste made from heated fruit is used to treat ringworm [45].

7. Some chemical compounds isolated from *Solanum torvum*

Solanum torvum contains a variety of bioactive compounds that give it its multiple pharmacological properties. As reported in reference studies [48–50], the chemical compounds identified in this plant and studied for their biological effects are: isoflavonoid sulfate and antiviral steroidal glycosides, torvanol A (a new isoflavonoid sulfate), torvoside H (a new steroidal glycoside), torvoside A (a previously recognized glycoside) and a tocopherol, solanolactosides A and B, and two newspirostanol glycosides (torvosides M and N). Certain structures have been identified, namely, solanolide 6-O-[a-l-rhamnopyranosyl-(1 → 3)-O-ß-d-quinovopyranoside], solanolide 6-O-[ß-d-xylopyranosyl-(1 → 3)-O-ß-d-quinovopyranoside], yamogenin 3-O-[ß-dglucopyranosyl-(1 → 6)-O-ß-d-glucopyranoside], neochlorogenic acid 3-O-[ß-d-glucopyranosyl(1 → 6)-O-ß-d-glucopyranoside], and so forth (**Figure 1**).

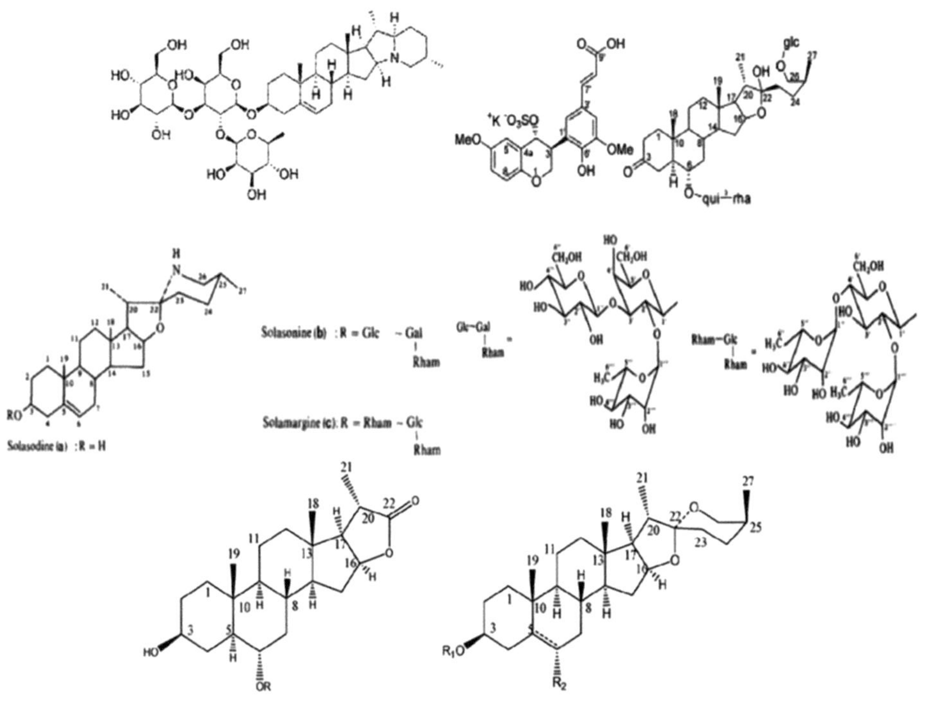

1 R=α-L-Rha(1→3)-*O*-β-D-Qui-
2 R=β-D-Xyl(1→3)-*O*-β-D-Qui-

3 Δ^5 R_1= β-D-glu-(1→6)-*O*-β-D-glu- R_2= H
4 5α-H R_1=β-D-glu-(1→6)-*O*-β-D-glu- R_2= OH

Figure 1.
Some isolated compounds from Solanum torvum.

8. Materials and methods

8.1 Biological materials

The biological material consisted of powder from dried *Solanum torvum* fruit and strains of *Salmonella sp* of human origin (stool and/or urine).

8.2 Method for preparing the various plant extracts

The fruits of the plant were harvested, sorted, washed, and dried at room temperature in the laboratory for three weeks. They were then pulverized in a Retsch-SK100 type mill to obtain a vegetable powder. This powder was then used to prepare the various extracts. The 100% ethanolic extract was prepared by dissolving 100 g of the previous plant powder in 1 liter of distilled water in a blender for 5 minutes to obtain a homogenate [49]. This was then filtered and evaporated in a blender-type oven for three days at 50 °C to obtain the aqueous extract. The latter was then macerated in 300 mL of pure ethanol in a blender for 5 minutes, then left to stand to obtain a supernatant and a pellet. These were subsequently further separated and evaporated in a Blender oven for three days at 50 °C. The 100% ethanolic extract (Eth 100%) obtained was taken from the pellet. In parallel with the preparation of the 100% ethanolic extract, another extract, the 70% hydroethanolic extract, was prepared using the same procedure as above. The only difference is that the solvent used in this case is a mixture of ethanol and distilled water (70/30, v/v). Final preparation of this extract yielded the 70% hydroethanol extract (HydroEth 70%). The resulting 100% ethanolic (Eth 100%) and 70% hydroethanolic (HydroEth 70%) extracts were stored separately in hermetically sealed jars and stored at room temperature for future testing.

8.3 Extraction yield calculation method

It was based on the method described by reference studies [18, 50, 51]. Yield is the quantity of extract obtained from a plant material. It is expressed as a percentage of dry matter (plant powder) and was calculated using the following formula:

$$R(\%) = M_1 \text{ x } 100 / M_0$$

- R: Yield of extract expressed as a percentage (%),
- M_1: Mass of extract (in g),
- M_0: Mass of vegetable powder (in g).

8.4 Method for evaluating the *in vitro* antibacterial activity of various *Solanum torvum* extracts

8.4.1 Method for preparing concentration ranges

This was achieved by dissolving 1 g of a previously prepared extract in 10 mL of distilled water to give an initial concentration of 100 mg/mL (tube 1 = T1). Concentrations in the other tubes (T2 to T6) were prepared from tube 1 (T1) using the liquid double dilution technique. To do this, a volume of 5 mL of sterile distilled water was distributed from T2 to T6. Next, a 5 mL volume of T1 was withdrawn, diluted with T2 and homogenized. This operation was repeated until T6. From T6 onward, the excess was discarded. Concentration ranges oscillated between 100 mg/mL and 3.125 mg/mL from T1 to T6.

8.4.2 Agar diffusion sensitivity test method

In this step, the bacterial inoculum was prepared from 1–2 colonies of *Salmonella sp*. These were then diluted in 0.85 NaCl solution and homogenized to obtain a 0.5 Mc Farland caliber. Next, an accurate Muller-Hinton (MH) agar plate was inoculated with the inoculum previously prepared by swabbing. Wells were subsequently drilled into the inoculated agar using a Pasteur pipette. Each well was filled with a given concentration of the initially prepared extract. It was also incubated for 18 to 24 hours at 37 °C. After this incubation time, diffusion of each concentration was used to delimit a zone of bacterial growth inhibition in the seeded agar plate. Finally, the inhibition diameter was measured to determine whether the bacterial strain tested was sensitive or resistant to the extract used. This agar diffusion method is useful for assessing the bacterial activity of different extracts [52].

8.4.3 Dilution sensitivity test method

8.4.3.1 Method for preparing inoculated broth

It was performed using 2 young *Salmonella sp* colonies aged 18 to 24 hours. Colonies were picked from the agar plate, mixed with a platinum loop in 10 mL of MH broth and incubated for 3 to 5 hours at 37 °C to obtain a pre-culture. Again, 0.1 mL of the pre-culture broth was removed and homogenized in a further 10 mL of MH broth to achieve an opalescence of 10^6 CFU/mL.

8.4.3.2 Method for determining Minimum Inhibitory Concentration (MIC)

This was achieved by taking 1.8 mL of the previously prepared *Salmonella sp* inoculated broth and transferring it into 7 tubes to form the experimental series. Within the experimental series, a volume of 0.2 mL of each concentration of initial extract prepared was placed separately in 6 tubes. The 7th tube was the growth control tube, to which 0.2 mL of sterile distilled water was added. Thus, the final volume in the 7 tubes of the experimental series was 2 mL. All were then incubated at 37 °C for 18 to 24 hours. After this incubation time, the MIC was determined by identifying the absence of turbidity with the naked eye and in daylight. The MIC corresponds to the lowest concentration of a compound or substance capable of inhibiting bacterial growth. It is given by the concentration of the first tube in which the culture is not turbid [22, 53].

8.4.3.3 Bacterial count method

This was carried out by diluting the bacterial culture in the growth control tube, preincubated at 37 °C for 18 to 24 hours (7th tube), from 10 to 10 down to 10^{-4}. Each dilution was then streaked 5 cm apart with a 2 µL calibrated platinum loop onto an MH agar plate (Box A). The plate was also incubated for 18 to 24 hours at 37 °C. After this time, Box A was used to determine the minimum bactericidal concentration.

8.4.3.4 Method for determining Minimum Bactericidal Concentration (MBC)

This involved inoculating each *Salmonella sp* culture from the experimental series separately on a 5 cm streak using a 2 µL calibrated platinum loop on a MH agar plate (Box B). It was followed by incubation at 37 °C for 18 to 24 hours. After this incubation period, the MBC was determined by comparing the number of *Salmonella sp* colonies on the various streaks on the B plate with those on the 10^{-4} dilution of the A plate. Indeed, according to reference studies [22, 54], the determination of the minimum bactericidal concentration (MBC) is possible by looking for the concentration leaving at most 0.01% surviving bacteria. However, according to reference [53]:

- if the MBC/MIC ratio ≤ 4, the substance tested is bactericidal.
- if the ratio MBC/MIC $^{>}$ 4, the substance tested is bacteriostatic.

DOI: http://dx.doi.org/10.5772/intechopen.1012825

8.5 Chemical test method for *Solanum torvum* fruit extracts

8.5.1 Qualitative analysis

They consisted in identifying compounds such as:

- polyphenols by reaction with ferric chloride ($FeCl_3$),
- flavonoids using the chloride vanillin and ammonia tests,
- coumarins with 96% ethanol, 10% NaoH and concentrated HCl,
- tannins with 80% methanol and 10% $FeCl_3$,
- saponosides with the foam test.

8.5.2 Quantitative analysis

8.5.2.1 Determination of total phenols

It was carried out using the Folin–Ciocalteu method, which is based on the redox reaction.

8.5.2.2 Determination of condensed tannins

It was tested using the vanillin method with HCl.

8.5.2.3 Total flavonoid content

It was produced using the colorimetric method with aluminum trichloride ($AlCl_3$).

8.5.2.4 Method for assessing the antioxidant activity of Solanum torvum fruit extracts using the DPPH test

It is based on a compound's ability to reduce the DPPH (2,2-diphenyl-1-picrylhydrazyl) radical.

9. Results

9.1 Yield of different extracts

The yield of the Eth 100% extract was 13.94%, while that of the HydroEth 70% extract was 5.64%. Thus, the yield of the Eth 100% extract was just over 2 times greater (13.94/5.64) than that of the HydroEth 70% extract.

9.2 Agar diffusion sensitivity tests

The results of agar diffusion sensitivity tests gave inhibition diameters of 9 mm for Eth 100% extract and 10 mm for HydroEth 70% extract. According to reference studies [55, 56], a bacterium is said to be:

- resistant to a plant extract when the inhibition diameter described around this extract is less than or equal to 8 mm,
- sensitive, if it is between 9 and 14 mm,
- very sensitive when it is between 15 and 19 mm,
- extremely sensitive when the diameter is greater than or equal to 20 mm.

9.3 Dilution sensitivity tests for MIC and MBC determination

The results of sensitivity tests using the dilution method yielded minimum inhibitory concentrations (MIC) of:

- 12.5 mg/mL of HydroEth 70% extract,
- 50 mg/mL of Eth 100% extract.

Similarly, these results enabled us to determine minimum bactericidal concentrations (MBC) of:

- 25 mg/mL of HydroEth 70% extract,
- 50 mg/mL of Eth 100% extract.

The MBC/MIC ratio gave a value of:

- 2 for HydroEth 70% extract,
- 1 for Eth 100% extract.

9.4 Chemical testing of *Solanum torvum* fruit extracts

The results of qualitative analyses of both extracts showed the presence of phytocompounds such as polyphenols, tannins, flavonoids, coumarins, and saponosides. Quantitative analyses yielded:

- 151.15 ± 0.95 mgEAG/gMS total phenols,
- 18.24 ± 1.31 mgEC/gMS condensed tannins,
- 88.37 ± 1.13 mgEQ/gMS total flavonoids in Eth 100% extract.
- 92.99 ± 2.9 mgEAG/gMS total phenols,
- 9.42 ± 1.63 mgEC/gMS condensed tannins,
- 49.11 ± 0.3 mgEQ/gMS total flavonoids in HydroEth 70% extract.

9.5 Evaluation of the antioxidant activity of *Solanum torvum* fruit extracts using the DPPH test

Results for the anti-free radical activity of vitamin C, Eth 100% extract, and HydroEth 70% extract yielded IC_{50} values of 0.007, 0.39, and 0.36 mg/mL, respectively.

10. Discussion

10.1 Yield of different extracts

The results of the yield calculation show that the Eth 100% extract is just over 2 times higher (13.94/5.64) than the HydroEth 70% extract. This may be justified by the fact that the extraction of bioactive substances may depend on the solvent and method used. So, water can isolate certain compounds such as polypeptides, lectins, starches, saponins, terpenes, and so forth, while ethanol can help reveal propolis, alkaloids, flavonoids, sterols, and so on [22, 57]. In terms of method, it should be noted that the aqueous extract served as the basis for the preparation of the Eth 100% extract. Subsequently, the Eth 100% extract could contain both substances soluble in both solvents (water and pure ethanol) and those specifically extractable with one of the solvents. These explanations could account for the high presence of the various compounds mentioned above and influence yield. In contrast, the HydroEth 70% extract can only isolate substances with solubility intermediate between ethanol and water.

10.2 Agar diffusion sensitivity tests

Inhibition diameters were 10 mm for the HydroEth 70% extract and 9 mm for the Eth 100% extract on *Salmonella sp* at a concentration of 100 mg/mL. These results demonstrate that *Salmonella sp* is sensitive to these two extracts, as their inhibition diameters ranged from 9 to 14 mm.

10.3 Dilution sensitivity tests for MIC and MBC determination

Antibacterial parameters (MIC and MBC) for the HydroEth 70% extract were 12.5 and 25 mg/mL, respectively, and the MBC/MIC ratio was 2. Similarly, the MBC/MIC ratio was 2. In the same vein, the Eth 100% extract produced an identical MIC and MBC value of 50 mg/mL. In addition, the MBC/MIC ratio was 1. These results thus confirm that both extracts are bactericidal on *Salmonella sp*, but with a higher bactericidal effect for the HydroEth 70% extract. Previous work by reference [58] on Eth extract from 100% of *Solanum torvum* leaves revealed bactericidal activity against *Salmonella sp*. These two results confirm that whatever the *Solanum torvum* organ used, antibacterial activity against *Salmonella sp* is observed.

10.4 Chemical testing of *Solanum torvum* fruit extracts

Qualitative analysis of both extracts revealed the presence of polyphenols, tannins, flavonoids, coumarins, and saponosides. These results are in line with those of reference [59] on *Solanum torvum* fruits. In the course of their work, these authors showed that *Solanum torvum* fruits contained alkaloids, and so on, in addition to the aforementioned compounds. Furthermore, the work of reference studies [56, 60, 61] stipulates that these bioactive substances possess antibacterial activities. Quantitative analysis revealed that both extracts contained varying levels of total polyphenols, flavonoids, and tannins. For the Eth 100% extract, the respective contents of total phenols, tannins, and flavonoids were 151.15 ± 0.95 mgEAG/gMS, 18.24 ± 1.31 mgEC/gMS, and 88.37 ± 1.13 mgEQ/gMS. For the HydroEth 70% extract, the respective contents of these same compounds were 92.99 ± 2.9 mgEAG/gMS, 9.42 ± 1.63 mgEC/gMS, and 49.11 ± 0.3 mgEQ/gMS. These results generally show a higher abundance of these compounds in the Eth 100% extract than in the HydroEth 70% extract. Nevertheless, the work of reference [57] on several medicinal plants has revealed that water is capable of isolating anthocyanins, tannins, saponins, terpenes, flavonols, and so forth. In the same way, this author showed that ethanol can highlight compounds such as tannins, polyphenols, polyacetylenes, flavonoids, sterols, alkaloids, propolis, and so on. Thus, during his work, the author revealed that ethanol can extract more bioactive substances than water. Consequently, the combination of these two solvents (water and ethanol) can extract a variety of bioactive molecules that are soluble in both water and ethanol, such as anthocyanins, tannins, saponins, terpenes, flavonols, polyphenols, polyacetylenes, flavonoids, sterols, alkaloids, propolis, and so forth. Therefore, the synergy of the bioactive substances that can be isolated by the water-ethanol mixture could justify the greater activity of the HydroEth 70% extract compared to Eth 100%, even though the compounds identified in this study are not present in high concentrations in this extract. In the same way, reference studies [62, 63] have established that these compounds possess anti-inflammatory, antibacterial, antiviral, antiallergic, antithrombotic, and vasodilatory activities. These results would justify the use of *Solanum torvum* in the treatment of antibacterial infections. Reference studies [51, 64] also highlighted the antibacterial activity of *Solanum torvum* fruit extracts on susceptible and resistant bacteria. Also, studies by reference [65] showed that the aqueous extract of *Solanum torvum* would possess antidiarrheal activities.

10.5 DPPH test

The anti-free radical activity results of the DPPH test for vitamin C, HydroEth 70%, and Eth 100% extracts gave IC_{50} values of 0.007, 0.36, and 0.39 mg/mL, respectively. These values correspond to the concentration of the substance required to inhibit 50% of free radicals in an antioxidant test. Therefore, the lower the value, the greater the anti-free radical activity. Consequently, vitamin C (positive control or reference) inhibited more than 51 (0.36/0.007) and 57 (0.39/0.007) times more free radicals in the medium than HydroEth 70% extract and Eth 100% extract, respectively. However, the HydroEth 70% and Eth 100% extracts show good anti-free radical activity, as they are still aggregates of molecules (polyphenols, tannins, flavonoids, coumarins, and saponosides), unlike the reference control (vitamin C, pure molecule). This work is in line with that of reference [48] when testing the ethanolic extract of *Solanum torvum* fruits.

11. Conclusion

This study revealed that the 100% ethanolic and 70% hydroethanolic extracts of *Solanum torvum* fruits had antibacterial activity against *Salmonella sp*. It showed that extraction with pure ethanol concentrated more bioactive substances than hydroethanolic extraction. These compounds are essentially polyphenols, tannins, flavonoids, coumarins, and saponosides. Of these, secondary metabolites, total phenols and flavonoids, and the condensed tannins measured had anti-free radical properties. Nevertheless, sensitivity tests in solid and liquid media showed that the hydroethanol extract was more bactericidal on *Salmonella sp* than the ethanol extract. The bactericidal effect observed was generally dose-dependent, since it depended on the concentration used. The fruits of *Solanum torvum* (a food plant) could therefore be used to develop a phytomedicine for the treatment of salmonellosis.

Author details

Obou Constantin Okou* and Margery Claude-Charlène Keke
Group of Excellence for Research into Traditional Pharmacopoeia Products (GeRTPhaPro), Agrovalorisation Laboratory, Agroforestry TRU, University of Jean Lorougnon Guede, Daloa, Côte d'Ivoire

*Address all correspondence to: constinokob@gmail.com

References

[1] Zrardi ME. Enterobacteriaceae: Epidemiology and Antibiotic Resistance. Algérie: Master of Molecular Biology of Microorganisms, Frères Mentouri Constantine University; 2020. 40 p

[2] Prével R. Mechanisms of dissemination of extended-spectrum beta-lactamase-producing Enterobacteriaceae in intensive care medicine. Doctoral thesis in Microbiology-Immunology. France: University of Bordeaux; 2021. 181 p. Available from: https://theses.hal.science/tel-03473742v1/file/PREVEL_RENAUD_2019_CORR.pdf

[3] Joly B, Reynaud A. Enterobacteriaceae: Systematics and diagnostic methods. Te Edition. 2007:3-182

[4] Bentabet J. Epidemiological profile of extended-spectrum B-lactamase-producing Enterobacteriaceae in hospitals Ibn Tofail [doctoral thesis]. Marrakech: University of Cadi Ayyad; 2021. 74 p

[5] Maddi SN, Menasra L. Enterobacterial Infections and their Antibiotic Resistance at the EPH d'El Khroub, Constantine. Algérie: Master of Microbiology and Hospital Hygiene, Frères Mentouri Constantine I University; 2022. p. 76. Available from: https://fac.umc.edu.dz/snv/bibliotheque/biblio/mmf/2022/Les%20infections%20%C3%A0%20ent%C3%A9robact%C3%A9ries%20et%20leurs%20antibior%C3%A9sistances%20au%20niveau%20de%20l%E2%80%99EPH%20d%E2%80%99El%20khroub,%20Constantine.pdf

[6] Iabadene H, Messai Y, Alouache S, Arlet G, Bakour R. Mechanisms of β-lactam and quinolone resistance in Enterobacter in Algiers hospitals. Review of Infectiology in Tunisia. 2010;**4**:24 p

[7] Gadou V. Molecular epidemiology of extended-spectrum β-lactamase-producing enterobacteria resistant to aminoglycosides and fluoroquinolones in Abidjan district, Côte d'Ivoire. Doctoral thesis in Functional and Molecular Biology. Abidjan, Côte d'Ivoire: University of Félix Houphouët-Boigny; 2019. 152 p. Availabe from: https://theses.hal.science/tel-02417084v1/file/Th%C3%A8se_GADOU%20Victoire.pdf

[8] Masterton R, Drusano G, Paterson DL, Park G. Appropriate antimicrobial treatment in nosocomial infections-the clinical challenges. Journal of Hospital Infection. 2003;**55**(Suppl 1):1-12

[9] Mangambu MJ, Mushagalusa KF, Kadima NJ. Photochemical study of some anti-diabetic medicinal plants from the town of Bukavu and surrounding area (South Kivu, R.D.Congo). Journal of Applied Biosciences. 2014;**75**:6211-6220

[10] Moroh J-LA. Bacterial resistance and antimicrobial phytomolecules from *Morinda morindoides*. Doctoral thesis in Microbiology-Biochemistry. France; Abidjan, Côte D'ivoire: Universities of Bretagne Occidentale; Felix Houphouët-Boigny; 2013. 204 p. Available from: https://theses.hal.science/tel-00935393v1

[11] Gueye F. Traditional Senegalese medicine: Examples of some medicinal plants from the traditional Senegalese Pharmacopoeia [doctoral thesis]. France: Marseille Faculty of Pharmacy, University of'Aix-Marseille; 2019. 176 p. Available from: https://dumas.ccsd.cnrs.fr/dumas-02351024v1

[12] Ouro-Djeri H, Koudouvo K, Tchacondo T, Ouro-Djeri E, Batawila K. Ethnobotanical and ethnopharmacological study of plants with therapeutic potential in Gboto and Esse-Godjin, two riverside townships in Togodo-Sud National Park (Yoto 3 commune), Togo. Ecosystem and Farmer Magazine. 2022;**2**(2):128-144. Available from: https://lbev-univlome.com/wp-content/uploads/2022/12/Ouro-Djeri-et-al.pdf

[13] Keirungi J, Fabricius C. Selecting medicinal plants for cultivation at Nqabara on the Eastern Cape Wild Coast, South Africa. South African Journal of Science. 2005;**101**:497-501

[14] Lahsissene H, Kahouadji A, Tijane M, Hseini S. Catalog of medicinal plants used in the zaër region, western Morocco. Lejeunia. Botanical Magazine. 2009;**186**:1-30. Available from: http://popups.ulg.ac.be/0457-4184

[15] Houmenou V, Adjatin A, Tossou MG, Yedomonhan H, Alexandre D, Gbenou J, et al. Ethnobotanical study of plants used in the treatment of female sterility in the departments of Ouémé and Plateau in southern Benin. International Journal of Biological and Chemical Sciences. 2017;**11**(4):1851-1871. Available from: https://agris.fao.org/search/en/providers/122414/records/6473afc12437ad1e5b938e98

[16] Candan F, Unlu M, Tepe B, Daferera D, Polissiou M, Sökmen A, et al. Antioxidant and antimicrobial activity of the essential oil and methanol extracts of *Achillea millefolium* subsp. *millefolium* Afan. (Asteraceae). Journal of Ethnopharmacology. 2003;**87**(2-3):215-220. DOI: 10.1016/s0378-8741(03)00149-1

[17] Lagnika L, Amoussa M, Adjovi Y, Sanni A. Antifungal, antibacterial and antioxidant properties of *Adansonia digitata* and *Vitex doniana* from Bénin pharmacopeia. Journal of Pharmacognosy and Phytotherapy. 2012;**4**(4):44-52

[18] Dinzedi MR. Antibacterial activity of *Terminalia catappa* and *Thonningia sanguinea* extracts on multi-resistant *Escherichia coli*, *Klebsiella pneumoniae* and *Staphylococcus aureus* of human origin. Doctoral thesis in Pharmacology of Natural Substances. Abidjan, Côte d'Ivoire: Option: Biochemistry Microbiology, University of Félix Houphouët-Boigny; 2015. 133 p

[19] Okou OC, Yapo Sopie E-S. Antibacterial Activity of *Solanum torvum* Leaves: Extracts of *Solanum torvum* leaves (Solanaceae) on the *In Vitro* Growth of 3 Strains of Enterobacteria. Berlin (Germany): European University Publishing; 2018. pp. 1-43. Available from:https://www.amazon.fr/Activit%C3%A9-antibact%C3%A9rienne-extraits-feuilles-Solanum/dp/6202272708

[20] Okou OC, Yayé YG, Ackah JAAB, Hamed D, Djaman AJ. *In vivo* action of *Mucuna pruriens* and *Millettia pinnata* (Fabaceae) minerals on the biochemical parameters of *Oryctolagus cuniculus*. International Journal of Applied Science Research. 2021;**4**(3):9-21

[21] Béné K, Camara D, Fofie NBY, Kanga Y, Yapi AB, Yapo YC, et al. Ethnobotanical study of medicinal plants used in the Transua department, Zanzan District (Côte d'Ivoire). Journal of Animal and Plant Sciences. 2016;**27**(2):4230-4250. Available from: https://m.elewa.org/JAPS/2015/27.2/2.bene.pdf

[22] Okou OC. Efficacy and spectrum of activity of extracts of *Mitracarpus scaber*

Zucc. Ex Schult+ Scult.f. (Rubiaceae) and fusidic acid on Gram-positive Cocci bacteria. Doctoral thesis in Biochemistry-Pharmacology. Abidjan, Côte d'Ivoire: University of Félix Houphouët-Boigny; 2012. 229 p. Available from: https://theses.hal.science/tel-02417073v1

[23] Henry I. Analytical epidemiology of *Salmonella subsp. enterica* and *Campylobacter spp*. in broiler farms on Reunion Island. Investigation of infectious sources of *Salmonella subsp. enterica* from production to processing. Doctoral thesis in Microbiology, Epidemiology and Veterinary Public Health. France: University of Réunion; 2011. 256 p. Available from: https://agritrop.cirad.fr/562952/

[24] Malle A. Surveillance of antimicrobial resistance in Salmonella strains isolated at the Rodolphe Mérieux Laboratory from 2015 to 2017 in Bamako, Mali [doctoral thesis]. Mali: Faculty of Pharmacy, University of Sciences, Techniques and Technologies of Bamako; 2018. 116 p. Available from: https://bibliosante.ml/handle/123456789/13250

[25] Aubry P, Gaüzère B-A. Salmonellosis, News 2021. Tropical Medicine. 2021. 19 p. Available from: http://www.medecinetropicale.com/

[26] Metuor DA. Molecular and kinetic characterization of extended-spectrum ß-lactamase (ESBL) types in bacterial strains collected at the Centre Hospitalier Universitaire Pédiatrique Charles De Gaulle (CHUP-CDG) in Ouagadougou [doctoral thesis]. Burkina Faso: Applied Sciences Specialty: Molecular Biology/Enzymology, University of Ouagadougou; 2014. 129 p

[27] Muller A. Proper use of antibiotics: Results of actions in different types of healthcare establishments. Doctoral Thesis in Life and Health Sciences. Franche-Comte, France: University of Bourgogne; 2017. 193 p. Available from: https://theses.hal.science/tel-01842246v1

[28] Mirabaud MI. Extended-spectrum beta-lactamase Enterobacteriaceae in pediatrics in 1996. Doctor of Medicine thesis. Suisse: University of Genève; 2003. 52 p. Available from: https://archive-ouverte.unige.ch/unige:173

[29] Debabza M. Emergence in hospitals of Gram-negative bacilli multiresistant to antibiotics: A bacteriological and molecular study. Doctoral thesis in Applied Microbiology. Algeria: Faculty of Science, University of Badji Mokhtar-Annaba; 2015. 217 p. Available from: https://dspace.univ-annaba.dz/items/31632c73-17c6-4e7a-ab24-1979be144385

[30] Sadikalay S. Influence of human and animal discharges on the spread of antibiotic resistance to humans, animals and the environment in Guadeloupe. Doctoral thesis in Microbiology. Guadeloupe, France: Faculty of Exact and Natural Sciences, University of the Antilles; 2018. 202 p. Available from: https://theses.fr/2018ANTI0251

[31] Hofer U. The cost of antimicrobial resistance. Nature Reviews. Microbiology. 2019;**17**(1):3-3. DOI: 10.1038/s41579-018-0125-x

[32] Gravey F. Genomics of multi-antibiotic-resistant bacteria in Normandia epidemic investigations, population studies, antibiotic resistance mechanisms. Doctoral Thesis, Life and Health Sciences. France: University of Caen Normandie; 2022. 197 p. Available from: https://theses.hal.science/tel-04128969v1

[33] Picot S, Rakotomalala RS, Farny K, Simac C, Michault A. Evolution of resistance to antibiotics from

1997 to 2005 in the Reunion Island. Médecine et Maladies Infectieuses. 2010;**40**(11):617-624

[34] Ahanogbe KAL. Bacterial resistance in diabetic wound infections: Diagnosis and monitoring at the Rodolphe Mérieux laboratory in Bamako [Doctoral thesis]. Mali: Faculty of Pharmacy, University of Sciences, Techniques and Technologies of Bamako; 2014 78 p. Available from: https://www.bibliosante.ml/bitstream/handle/123456789/1028/14P23.pdf?sequence=1&isAllowed=y

[35] Elouennass M, Sahnoun I, Zrara A, Bajjou T, Elhamzaoui S. Epidemiology and susceptibility profile of blood culture isolates in an intensive care unit (2002-2005). Medicine and Infectious Diseases. 2008;**38**(1):18-24

[36] OMS. Regional strategy to accelerate the implementation and monitoring of national action plans to combat antimicrobial resistance (2023-2030) in the WHO African Region. In: Seventy-Third Session Gaborone, Republic of Botswana, August 28–September 1, 2023. 2023. 9 p. Available from:https://iris.who.int/bitstream/handle/10665/373260/AFR-RC73-6-fre.pdf?sequence=1&isAllowed=y

[37] Guillaumy L. Antibiotic resistance in West Africa: Emergence, struggles and challenges [Doctoral thesis]. France: Marseille Faculty of Pharmacy, University of'Aix-Marseille; 2024. 114 p. Available from:https://dumas.ccsd.cnrs.fr/dumas-04643328v1/file/The%CC%80se%20Lucie%20Guillaumy.pdf

[38] Jouzier E. Medicinal Solanaceae and philately. Bulletin of the Pharmacy Society of Bordeaux. 2005;**144**:311-332. Available from: https://www.socpharmbordeauxasso.fr/pdf/pdf-144/144-311-332.pdf

[39] Telefo PB, Lienou LL, Yemele MD, Lemfack MC, Mouokeu C. Ethnopharmacological survey of plants used for the treatment of female infertility in Baham, Camroom. Journal of Ethnopharmacology. 2011;**136**:178-187

[40] Jiofack T, Ayissi L, Fokunang C, Guedje N, Kemeuze V. Ethnobotany and phytomedicine of the upper Nyong valley forest in Cameroon. African Journal of Pharmacy and Pharmacology. 2009;**3**(4):144-150

[41] OOAS (Organisation Ouest Africaine de la Santé). West African Pharmacopoeia. In: *Solanum Torvum*. 2013. 195-198 pp

[42] Agyare C, Asase A, Lechtenberg M, Niehues M, Deters A, Hensel A. An ethnopharmacological survey and *in vitro* confirmation of ethnopharmacological use of medicinal plants used for wound healing in Bosomtwi-Atwima-Kwanwoma area, Ghana. Journal of Ethnopharmacology. 2009;**125**:393-403. DOI: 10.1016/j.jep.2009.07.024

[43] Amujoyegbe OO, Idu M, Agbedahunsi JM, Erhabor JO. Ethnomedicinal survey of medicinal plants used in the management of sickle cell disorder in Southern Nigeria. Journal of Ethnopharmacology. 2016;**185**:347-360. DOI: 10.1016/j.jep.2016.03.042

[44] N'guessan K, Kouassi KH, Ouattara D. Plants used to treat anaemia, in traditional medicine, by Abbey and Krobou populations, in the South of Côte-d'Ivoire. Journal of Applied Sciences Research. 2010;**6**(8):1291-1297

[45] Nicolas JP. Medicinal Plants from Northern Madagascar Antakarana Ethnobotany and Scientific Information, *Solanum torvum* Sw. rue saint Michel (France): Jardins du monde; 2012. p. 240. Available from:https://www.

ethnopharmacologia.org/prelude2020/pdf/biblio-hn-42-nicolas.pdf

[46] Yuanyuan L, Jianguang L, Xuefeng H, Lingyi K. Four new steroidal glycosides from *Solanum torvum* and their cytotoxic activities. Steroids. 2009;**74**:95-101

[47] Zubaida Y, Ying W, Elias B. Phytochemistry and Pharmacological Studies on *Solanum torvum* Swartz. Journal of Applied Pharmaceutical Science. 2013;**3**(04):152-160. DOI: 10.7324/JAPS.2013.3428

[48] Pandey G, Prajapati KK, Pandey R. Distribution, Taxonomy and Medicinal Importance of *Solanum torvum* Sw. Phyto Talks. 2024;**2**:95-105

[49] Zirihi GN, Grenier P, Guédé-Guina F, Bodo B, Mambu L. Isolation, characterization and antiplasmodial activity of steroidal alkaloids from *Funtumia elastica* (Preuss) Stapf. Bioorganic and Medicinal Chemistry Letters. 2005;**15**:2637-2640

[50] Bssaibis F, Gmira N, Meziane M. Antibacterial activity of *Dittrichia viscosa* (L.) W. Greuter. Review of Industrial. Sanitary and Environmental Microbiology. 2009;**3**:44-55

[51] Okou OC, Yapo SE-S, Kouassi KC, Komenan NR, Monthaut SV, Kra AKM, et al. Evaluation of the antibacterial activity of fruit extracts of *Solanum torvum* Swartz (Solanaceae) on the *in* vitro growth of seven (07) strains of enterobacteria with different profiles (resistant or susceptible). International Journal of Biological and Chemical Sciences. 2019;**13**(3):1510-1526

[52] Wiegand I, Hilpert K, Hancock REW. Agar and broth dilution methods to determine the minimal inhibitory concentration (MIC) of antimicrobial substances. Nature Protocols. 2007;**3**:163-175

[53] Marmonier AA. Introduction to antibiotic study techniques. In: Medical Bacteriology. Paris, France: Standard Techniques. Doin; 1990. pp. 227-236

[54] Sirot J. Evaluating the anti-bacterial activity of antibiotics *in vitro*. In: Medical Bacteriology. 2nd ed. Flammarion; 1990. pp. 297-315

[55] Ponce A, Fritz R, Der Vall C, Roura S. Antimicrobial activity of essential oils on the native microflora of organic swiss chard. Society of Food Science and Technology. 2003;**36**:679-684

[56] Atsain MR. Phytochemical, microbiological and antioxidant investigations of extracts from organs of *Schrankia leptocarpa* d.c (Mimosaceae). Doctoral thesis in Chemistry of Natural Substances/Microbiology. Abidjan, Côte d'Ivoire: University of Nangui Abrogoua; 2017. 150 p

[57] Cowan MM. Plants products as antimicrobial agents. Clinical Microbiology Reviews. 1999;**12**(4):564-582

[58] Okou OC, Yapo SE-S, Kporou KE, Baibo GL, Monthaut S, Djaman AJ. Evaluation of the antibacterial activity of *Solanum torvum* Swartz (Solanaceae) leaf extracts on the *in vitro* growth of 3 strains of enterobacteria. Journal of Applied Biosciences. 2018;**122**:12287-12295

[59] Dan CG, Yao K, Koffi BL. Active ingredients and identification of sugars in *Solanum anguivi* lam and *Solanum torvum* eggplants harvested in Côte d'Ivoire. European Scientific Journal. 2021;**17**(21):33-45

[60] Morel S. Phytochemical study and biological evaluation of *Derris*

ferruginean Benth. (Fabaceae). Unique doctoral thesis, ANGERS Pharmaceutical Sciences and Health Engineering TRU. France: University of Angers; 2011. 263 p. Available from:https://theses.hal.science/tel-00671071v1

[61] Daglia M. Polyphenols as antimicrobial agents. Current Opinion in Biotechnology. 2012;**23**(2):174-181

[62] Gulcin I, Huyut Z, Elmastas M, Aboul-Enein HY. Radical scavenging and antioxidant activity of tannic acid. Arabian Journal of Chemistry. 2010;**3**(1):43-53

[63] Konan KF. Antibacterial activity against extended-spectrum beta-lactamase-producing Enterobacteriaceae, and *in vitro* antioxidant potential of *Terminalia glaucescens* planch ex Benth. (Combretaceae), a West African medicinal plant. Doctoral thesis, Biosciences TRU. Abidjan, Côte d'Ivoire: University of Félix Houphouët-Boigny; 2015. 121 p

[64] N'guessan KJ, Toty AA, Irié BJS, Konan KF, Guessennd N, Abo KJ-C. Antibacterial Properties of an Aqueous Extract of *Solanum torvum* (Solanaceae) on a Few Multidrug Resistant Bacterial Strains to Common Antibiotics. American Scientific Research Journal for Engineering, Technology, and Sciences. 2019;**54**(1):137-146

[65] N'guessan KJ, Irie BJS, Kahou BGP, Abo KJ-C. Antidiarrheal properties of the aqueous extract of *Solanum torvum* (Solanaceae) in the rat strain Wistar. European Scientific Journal. 2020;**16**(6):112-125

Section 4

Risk Analysis and Future Approaches

Chapter 9

Course Corrections Are Needed to Better Address the Risk of Salmonellosis from Poultry Food

Thomas P. Oscar

Abstract

Computer models that predict consumer exposure and response to *Salmonella* in poultry food are valuable tools for helping assess and manage this risk to public health. However, model predictions are only as good as the data and models used to make them. If the data and models are inaccurate, the model simulations and predictions will be erroneous, and the risk management decision will be wrong. In this study, a comparison is made between two different data collection and modeling methods for assessing the risk of salmonellosis from poultry food. First, are the probabilistic methods used in Quantitative Microbial Risk Assessment (QMRA). Second, are the rare event methods used in the Poultry Food Assess Risk Model (PFARM). Based on the comparison of these data collection and modeling methods and a case study, it was concluded that course corrections are needed to better assess and manage the risk of salmonellosis from poultry food. Namely, a shift away from the probabilistic methods of QMRA to the rare event methods of PFARM and a shift in focus from the pre-harvest and post-harvest sectors of the farm-to-table chain to the consumer sector where the most important risk factors for salmonellosis from poultry food are found.

Keywords: *Salmonella*, poultry food, risk assessment, public health, comparison, QMRA, PFARM

1. Introduction

A pathogen reduction, hazard analysis and critical control point, and performance standard (PR-HACCP-PS) program was implemented in the United States to reduce the risk of salmonellosis from poultry food [1]. This program has been successful at reducing *Salmonella* prevalence in carcass rinse aliquot samples at final product testing in the processing plant [2]. However, it has not been successful at reducing the risk or rate of foodborne salmonellosis. This has prompted a proposed expansion of the PR-HACCP-PS program to include new PS for *Salmonella* number and serotype [3].

When data collection and modeling methods for predicting the risk of salmonellosis from poultry food emerged in the 1990s there was a divergence of methods leading to an accepted approach (Quantitative Microbial Risk Assessment or QMRA) and an

 IntechOpen

alternative approach (Poultry Food Assess Risk Model or PFARM). Here, a comparison of QMRA and PFARM data collection and modeling methods is made with a brief description of key studies. To reduce self-citation of PFARM studies, five recent studies [4–8] that review why and how the PFARM data collection and modeling methods were developed and used will be emphasized.

2. Comparison of QMRA and PFARM

The quality of a computer model simulation and prediction is only as good as the data and models on which it is based. Thus, if the data collection and modeling methods are not accurate, the model simulations and predictions will not be accurate, and the resulting course of action will not be the right one. After the comparison of the data collection and modeling methods used in QMRA and PFARM, a case study will be presented to illustrate the importance of the differences in these two approaches to assessing the risk of salmonellosis from poultry food.

2.1 Sampling method

Salmonella may be unattached, attached, or entrapped in the poultry food matrix [9, 10]. Therefore, the sampling method used must be able to detect a single cell of viable *Salmonella* regardless of how it is associated with the poultry food matrix, or the prevalence, number, and serotype data will not be accurate.

QMRA - Rinsing (chicken carcass and parts) and swabbing (turkey carcass and parts) of poultry food recovers some but not all the *Salmonella* [11]. This leads to an underestimation of prevalence, number, and serotype, and an inaccurate simulation and prediction of the risk of salmonellosis. *PFARM* - Whole sample enrichment (WSE) detects more if not all *Salmonella* on and in poultry food leading to more accurate prevalence, number, and serotype data for simulating and predicting the risk of salmonellosis [8]. *Key QMRA study* - Simmons et al. [12] reported that 13% of chicken carcasses were positive for *Salmonella* when rinse samples were used, whereas 38% were positive for *Salmonella* when WSE was used. *Key PFARM study* - Parveen et al. [13] reported that *Salmonella* prevalence was 88% in a compliant commercial processing plant (i.e. < 9.8%) when chicken carcasses were sampled using WSE instead of the carcass rinse aliquot method.

2.2 *Salmonella* prevalence

QMRA- *Salmonella* prevalence of poultry food is not expressed and simulated as a function of the size of sample analyzed resulting in an inaccurate simulation and prediction of the risk of salmonellosis. *PFARM* - *Salmonella* prevalence is expressed and simulated as a function of the size of sample analyzed resulting in a more accurate simulation and prediction of the risk of salmonellosis from poultry food. *Key QMRA study* - Surkiewicz et al. [14] reported that *Salmonella* in rinse samples of chicken carcasses was 4.9% when 10 mL was examined and 20.5% when 270 mL was examined. Thus, it has been known for some time, since 1969, that *Salmonella* prevalence changes in a nonlinear manner as a function of the size of sample analyzed, yet, in QMRA it is expressed and simulated without a denominator. *Key PFARM study* - Oscar [8] reported that *Salmonella* prevalence increases in a nonlinear manner as a function of the size of poultry food sample analyzed.

2.3 Microbiological independence

QMRA - The split sample method uses a different sample and a different size sample of poultry food for *Salmonella* prevalence (cultural isolation) and number (most probable number or MPN) leading to inaccurate data for simulating and predicting the risk of salmonellosis because the microbiological independence of the samples is not recognized. *PFARM* - A single sample of poultry food is used for *Salmonella* prevalence (cultural isolation) and number (growth units), which is determined by WSE, real-time quantitative polymerase chain reaction (qPCR). This leads to more accurate data for simulating and predicting the risk of salmonellosis. *Key QMRA study* - Bemrah et al. [15] used the split sample method for prevalence and number of *Salmonella* in turkey cordon bleu. However, only 2 of 36 samples that tested positive for *Salmonella* by cultural isolation, tested positive in the MPN assay because a different sample and a much smaller sample was used to determine *Salmonella* number. *Key PFARM study* - Oscar [8] used the one pathogen cell test to show why the QMRA split sample method is inaccurate and the PFARM single sample method (WSE-qPCR) is more accurate.

2.4 Location of final product testing

QMRA – Final product testing for *Salmonella* is in the poultry food processing plant leading to an inaccurate simulation and prediction of the risk of salmonellosis because the growth and spread of *Salmonella* in packaged poultry food after processing leads to unpredictable changes in *Salmonella* serotype prevalence and number among servings in the package [16]. *PFARM* - Final product testing for *Salmonella* is at the start of meal preparation to better capture effects of poultry food production, processing, distribution, storage, and interventions on *Salmonella* serotype prevalence and number leading to a more accurate simulation and prediction of the risk of salmonellosis [8].

2.5 *Salmonella* number

QMRA - Results of the MPN assay used in the split sample method are expressed and simulated on a per gram basis resulting in an inaccurate simulation and prediction of the risk of salmonellosis from poultry food because *Salmonella* number does not increase in a linear manner as a function of serving size, which is assumed in this method of expression. *PFARM* – Results of the WSE-qPCR method used in the single sample method are expressed and simulated as a function of the size of sample analyzed resulting in more accurate simulation and prediction of the risk of salmonellosis from poultry food because *Salmonella* number is predicted to increase in a non-linear manner as a function of serving size. *Key QMRA study* - De Man [17] reported that for a 3 replicate by 3 dilution MPN assay, the MPN per g ranges from 0.3 for a result of 0-0-1 to 110 for a result of 3-3-2. However, when results are expressed as a function of the size of sample analyzed, the range is 1 to 366 MPN per 3.33 g, which is more accurate. The MPN result of 0-0-0 is not ≤ 0.3/g. Rather, it is 0 per 3.33 g or negative for *Salmonella*. *Key PFARM study* - Oscar [8] reported that *Salmonella* number increases in a nonlinear manner as a function of the size of sample analyzed or simulated.

2.6 Growth potential

QMRA - The MPN method does not capture the growth potential of *Salmonella*, which is important for accurate simulation and prediction of the risk of salmonellosis from poultry food because it captures the physiological state of the pathogen and the impact of the native microflora on its growth in the poultry food matrix. Importantly, it does not capture effects of processes that injure *Salmonella* and reduce the risk of salmonellosis from poultry food. *PFARM* – The WSE-qPCR method is a growth-based assay that captures the growth potential of *Salmonella* in poultry food resulting in a more accurate simulation and prediction of the risk of salmonellosis. *Key PFARM study* - Oscar [8] used WSE-qPCR to enumerate *Salmonella* growth units in poultry food as a non-linear function of serving size.

2.7 Exposure assessment

QMRA - The probabilistic method overestimates consumer exposure to *Salmonella* because it only simulates contaminated grams of poultry food and assumes that *Salmonella* number increases in a linear manner as a function of serving size. *PFARM* - The rare event modeling method does not overestimate consumer exposure to *Salmonella* because it simulates both contaminated and noncontaminated servings and predicts the non-linear increase of *Salmonella* prevalence and number as a function of serving size. *Key PFARM study* - Oscar [5] provided 13 reasons why the QMRA probabilistic method provides an inaccurate prediction of consumer exposure to *Salmonella* from poultry food.

2.8 Dose-response assessment

QMRA - The probabilistic, sigmoidal, dose-response model [18] and its variants [3] do not explicitly simulate the *Salmonella*, poultry food meal, and consumer interaction or disease triangle resulting in an inaccurate simulation and prediction of the risk of salmonellosis. *PFARM* - The rare event, disease triangle, dose-response model [6] simulates risk of salmonellosis as a function of the zoonotic potential of *Salmonella* serotypes, the buffering capacity of the poultry food meal, and the health and immunity of the consumer. *Key PFARM study* - Oscar [19] reported that the dose-response curve is non-sigmoid in shape when the food is contaminated with two or more serotypes of *Salmonella* with different virulence and prevalence.

2.9 Risk prediction

QMRA - Predicts that a reduction of *Salmonella* in poultry food at final product testing will result in like reduction in the risk of salmonellosis [3], which is not consistent with the current situation in the poultry food industry. *PFARM* - Predicts that a reduction of *Salmonella* in poultry food at final product testing will not result in like reduction in the risk of salmonellosis, which is consistent with the current situation in the poultry food industry. *Key PFARM study* - Oscar [20] showed that there was no relationship between *Salmonella* levels at final product testing and risk of salmonellosis because of post-testing risk factors.

2.9.1 Risk prediction adjustment

QMRA - A correction factor is needed to align predictions of the risk of salmonellosis from poultry food with epidemiological data [3]. *PFARM* - No correction factor is needed to align predictions of the risk of salmonellosis from poultry food with epidemiological data [20]. *Key PFARM study* - Oscar [5] provided 13 reasons why the probabilistic modeling method used in QMRA makes inaccurate predictions of the risk of salmonellosis from poultry food.

2.10 Lot size

QMRA - Individual grams of *Salmonella*-contaminated poultry food is simulated from final product testing until consumption. At consumption they are multiplied by serving size and initial *Salmonella* prevalence resulting in an inaccurate simulation and prediction of the risk of salmonellosis. This is because lot size increases at consumption as a function of mean serving size and initial *Salmonella* prevalence. Thus, the lot size could differ among scenarios resulting in confounded comparisons. *PFARM- Salmonella*-contaminated and non-contaminated servings and *Salmonella* serotype prevalence and number (growth units) per size of sample analyzed are simulated from final product testing to consumption for more accurate prediction of the risk of salmonellosis because lot size at final product testing and at consumption is the same resulting in non-confounded comparisons among scenarios [5].

2.11 Predictive models

Predictive models for cross-contamination, growth, and thermal death of *Salmonella* in poultry food are used in QMRA and PFARM for exposure assessment. However, important differences exist for how predictive models are used to predict the risk of salmonellosis from poultry food.

2.11.1 Cross-contamination

QMRA - *Salmonella* transfer rates from poultry food to kitchen fomites and then to ready-to-eat (RTE) food are used to simulate cross-contamination of RTE food with *Salmonella*, which is simulated as probabilistic event [21]. This method does not consider *Salmonella* as a minority member of the native microflora of food. *PFARM* - Bacterial transfer rates from poultry food to kitchen fomites and then to RTE food are used to simulate cross-contamination of RTE food with native microflora including *Salmonella*, whose transfer is simulated as a discrete event using the rare event, line of transfer method [5]. This method simulates *Salmonella* as a minority member of the native microflora leading to more accurate simulation and prediction of the risk of salmonellosis because in nature, a cell of *Salmonella* does not have a probability of transfer, rather, it is transferred or not.

2.11.2 Growth

QMRA- Models for growth of *Salmonella* are developed using a mixture of serotypes inoculated at a high and nonecological level in poultry food without native microflora resulting in a less accurate simulation and prediction of the growth of *Salmonella* and risk of salmonellosis [22]. *PFARM* - Models for growth of *Salmonella* are developed using individual serotypes inoculated at a low and ecological level in poultry food with native microflora leading to a more accurate simulation and prediction of the growth of *Salmonella* and the risk of salmonellosis [4]. *Key QMRA study* - Kim et al. [3] stated that serotype-specific growth models are needed for accurate risk assessment. *Key PFARM study* - Oscar [23] developed a model for three serotypes of *Salmonella* on poultry food for use in risk assessment.

2.11.3 Thermal death

QMRA – Models for thermal death of *Salmonella* are developed with a mixture of serotypes and a high and nonecological number of the pathogen in poultry food without native microflora [24]. In addition, the models predict the probability of *Salmonella* survival, which is >0 for all grams simulated [25]. This leads to an overestimation of consumer exposure to *Salmonella* and an inaccurate simulation and prediction of the risk of salmonellosis from cooked poultry food [5]. *PFARM* – Models for thermal death of *Salmonella* are developed with individual serotypes of *Salmonella* in poultry food with native microflora [26]. In addition, a rare event, line of death method is used to simulate survival of individual cells of *Salmonella* as minority members of the native microflora of poultry food during cooking [5]. Thus, survival of a *Salmonella* cell is simulated as a discrete (survival or no survival) event resulting in most (> 97%) cooked servings having zero *Salmonella* at consumption and the rest having ≥1 *Salmonella.* This leads to a more accurate simulation of what occurs in nature and a more accurate prediction of the risk of salmonellosis from cooked poultry food [5].

2.11.4 Model validation

QMRA- Models for behavior of *Salmonella* in poultry food are validated using conventional statistical methods and the bias and accuracy factor method of Ross [27]. These methods have no criteria for test data, limited criteria for model performance, and no criteria for model validation. This leads to an incomplete, less accurate, and more biased validation of models. In turn, this could lead to less accurate and more biased simulation and prediction of the risk of salmonellosis from poultry food. *PFARM* - Models for behavior of *Salmonella* in poultry food are validated using the Acceptable Prediction Zones (APZ) method [4]. The APZ method has objective criteria for test data, model performance, and model validation resulting in more accurate and less biased models and more accurate simulation and prediction of the risk of salmonellosis from poultry food. *Key PFARM study* - Oscar [7] provided 12 reasons why the APZ method is better than conventional methods and the bias and accuracy factor method of Ross for validating predictive models.

2.12 Case study

The end game of a program like PR-HACCP-PS is the identification and removal of unsafe lots of poultry food from the marketplace. However, the use of less accurate data and models increases identification of safe lots of poultry food as unsafe and unsafe lots of poultry food as safe. Both situations harm public health. The first by shortages, inflation, malnutrition, lower immunity, and more disease. The second by increased hospitalization and death and loss of brand confidence resulting in economic damage. Thus, it is important to get it right.

Data for *Salmonella* prevalence, number (growth units), and serotypes of chicken gizzards [8] were collected over time in a production chain using PFARM methods. The data was used to compare QMRA and PFARM modeling methods for predicting consumer exposure to *Salmonella* [5]. It was found that QMRA predicted higher consumer exposure to *Salmonella* than PFARM using the same data and exposure pathways [5].

In this case study, the comparison was extended to predicting risk of salmonellosis (illness) from chicken gizzards. However, the data was repurposed. Instead of five scenarios for running windows of 60 samples over time in the production chain, the five time-period scenarios represented five, 1000 kg lots of chicken gizzards.

2.12.1 Risk of salmonellosis among lots of chicken gizzards

QMRA: The risk of salmonellosis (illness) differed ($p \leq 0.05$) among lots of chicken gizzards (**Figure 1A**). It was highest for lots A and B, lowest for lot D, and intermediate and the same for lots C and E. *PFARM*: The risk of salmonellosis differed ($p \leq 0.05$) among lots of chicken gizzards (**Figure 1B**). It was higher for lot E than for lot B; otherwise, it was the same for all lots. Compared to QMRA (**Figure 1A**), the risk of salmonellosis predicted by PFARM (**Figure 1B**) was lower and differed less among lots. The results for QMRA were like those for exposure [5].

2.12.2 Risk of salmonellosis as a function of dose

QMRA- The probability of illness increased in an exponential manner as a function of the dose of *Salmonella* consumed from chicken gizzard meals (**Figure 2A**). This was because differences in zoonotic potential of *Salmonella*, buffering capacity of the meal, and consumer health and immunity were not explicitly simulated in the dose-response model. For the simulated replicate of lot E (**Figure 2A**), the probabilistic method used in the QMRA predicted 9–10 cases of salmonellosis per 1000 kg of chicken gizzards. In this case, all meals (n = 5952) had a *Salmonella* dose consumed that was >0. The meals with *Salmonella* doses >0 and < 1 were 5833, ≥ 1 and < 10 were 51, and ≥ 10 and < 10,000 were 68. However, the probabilistic modeling method used in QMRA does not provide an accurate simulation and prediction of what occurs in nature for the reasons stated above. In fact, it incorrectly mimicked consumer exposure to *Salmonella* [5] and resulted in a biased and overestimated prediction of the risk of salmonellosis. Moreover, it incorrectly simulated and predicted that a reduction in *Salmonella* dose consumed would result in a like reduction in the risk of salmonellosis, which is not what occurs in nature. Again, this occurred because

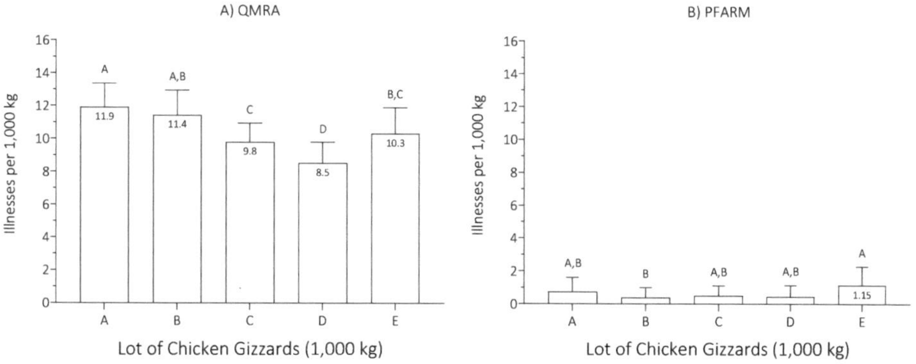

Figure 1.
Risk of salmonellosis (illness) from chicken gizzard meals as predicted by: (A) the probabilistic method of QMRA; and (B) the rare event method of PFARM for the same data and risk pathways. Bars are means ± standard deviation of 20 replicate simulations. The lot size simulated was 1000 kg of chicken gizzards per replicate simulation. The average portion size was 168 g per meal. Thus, 5952 meals were simulated. Within a panel, bars with different letters differ at p ≤ 0.05 *per one-way analysis of variance followed by Tukey's multiple comparison test (Prism, version 10, GraphPad Software, Boston, MA). Abbreviations: QMRA = quantitative microbial risk assessment; and PFARM = poultry food assess risk model.*

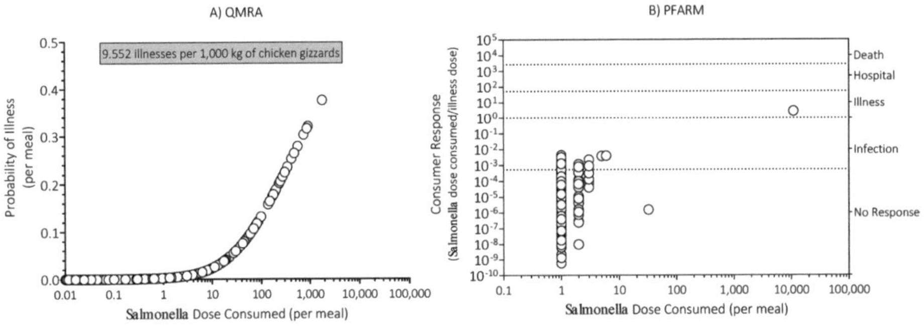

Figure 2.
The relationship between Salmonella *dose consumed from meals of chicken gizzards and (A) probability of illness or salmonellosis as predicted by QMRA and (B) consumer response as predicted by PFARM for a single replication from lot E. Abbreviations: QMRA = quantitative microbial risk assessment; and PFARM = poultry food assess risk model.*

the QMRA method did not explicitly simulate differences in zoonotic potential of *Salmonella*, buffering capacity of the meal, and consumer health and immunity.

PFARM - In contrast to QMRA, PFARM predicted that consumer response did not increase as a function of the *Salmonella* dose consumed from 1 to 100 growth units (**Figure 2B**). In fact, the consumer who ate the meal with 30 growth units had no response, whereas some consumers who ate meals with lower doses became infected (fecal shedding or antibody response with no symptoms of salmonellosis) with *Salmonella*. In contrast to QMRA, which predicted 9–10 cases of salmonellosis from lot E, PFARM only predicted one case (**Figure 2B**). In addition, PFARM predicted that most meals (5675 of 5952) resulted in no exposure to *Salmonella* and of those that resulted in exposure, most (275 of 277) had *Salmonella* doses from 1 to 10 growth units, whereas only two had a *Salmonella* dose >10 growth units. Thus, compared to QMRA (**Figure 2A**), PFARM (**Figure 2B**) predicted much less exposure to *Salmonella* and much less risk of salmonellosis. One important difference was the PFARM simulated the zoonotic potential of *Salmonella* serotypes, the buffering capacity of the meal, and the health and immunity of the consumer in its dose-response model, whereas QMRA did not [6].

2.13 Lessons learned from COVID-19 pandemic

A lesson learned from the coronavirus disease 2019 (COVID-19) pandemic was that zoonotic diseases can become endemic at a baseline level that fluctuates over time in response to changes in the pathogen, environment, and host interaction or disease triangle [28]. This same dynamic may be at play in salmonellosis from poultry food leading to the possibility that salmonellosis from poultry food may be at an endemic level that is fluctuating over time in response to changes in the disease triangle. Thus, it might be difficult to reduce foodborne salmonellosis further because a reduction in consumer exposure to *Salmonella* could be countered by a decrease in consumer immunity to salmonellosis. In other words, interventions like a PR-HACCP-PS program that reduce *Salmonella* at final product testing may have the unintended consequence of decreasing consumer immunity to salmonellosis [29] and help explain why PR-HACCP-PS has not reduced the risk of salmonellosis from poultry food.

Another lesson learned from the Covid-19 pandemic was that acquired immunity to the pathogen (severe acute respiratory syndrome coronavirus 2 or SARS-CoV-2) from vaccination or recent illness, reduces the risk of hospitalization and death [30]. Thus, in PFARM, the risk endpoint is severe salmonellosis (hospitalization, death) instead of salmonellosis (illness, hospitalization, death) because illness is viewed as important for maintaining consumer immunity to salmonellosis and reducing the risk of hospitalization and death.

Finally, a risk-to-risk comparison of the COVID-19 pandemic to salmonellosis from chicken indicates that it would take 1931 years for salmonellosis from chicken to cause the same number of hospitalizations as the COVID-19 pandemic and 18,073 years for salmonellosis from chicken to cause the same number of deaths as the COVID-19 pandemic [31, 32]. Thus, compared to COVID-19, salmonellosis from chicken poses a much lower risk to public health.

3. Conclusions

The comparison of QMRA and PFARM methods indicates that course corrections are needed to better address the risk of salmonellosis from poultry food. First, a shift from the probabilistic data collection and modeling methods used in QMRA to the rare event data collection and modeling methods used in PFARM is needed to better simulate and predict the risk of salmonellosis from poultry food. Second, a shift in focus from the pre-harvest and post-harvest sectors in QMRA to the consumer sector in PFARM is needed because the most important risk factors for salmonellosis are in the consumer sector. This would involve the application of PFARM data collection and modeling methods in the consumer sector to better identify lots of unsafe poultry food, if they exist. The PFARM methods could also be used to test the hypothesis that salmonellosis from poultry food is at a baseline level that cannot be reduced further.

Acknowledgements

The author thanks Vijay Juneja of the United States Department of Agriculture, Agricultural Research Service for his help in publishing this work. Mention of trade names or commercial products is solely for providing specific information and does not imply recommendation or endorsement by the United States Department of Agriculture, which is an equal opportunity provider and employer. The opinions expressed are those of the author and do not represent an official position of the United States Department of Agriculture.

Conflict of interest

The author declares no conflict of interest.

Author details

Thomas P. Oscar
United States Department of Agriculture, Agricultural Research Service, Microbial and Chemical Food Safety Research Unit, University of Maryland Eastern Shore Worksite, Princess Anne, Maryland, USA

*Address all correspondence to: thomas.oscar@usda.gov

References

[1] McNamara AM. Generic HACCP application in broiler slaughter and processing. Journal of Food Protection. 1997;**60**:579-604

[2] Williams MS, Ebel ED, Saini G, Nyirabahizi E. Changes in *Salmonella* contamination in meat and poultry since the introduction of the pathogen reduction and hazard analysis and critical control point rule. Journal of Food Protection. 2020;**83**(10):1707-1717. DOI: 10.4315/JFP-20-126

[3] Kim M, Barnett-Neefs C, Chavez RA, Kealey E, Wiedmann M, Stasiewicz MJ. Risk assessment predicts most of the salmonellosis risk in raw chicken parts is concentrated in those few products with high levels of high-virulence serotypes of *Salmonella*. Journal of Food Protection. 2024;**87**(7):100304. DOI: 10.1016/j.jfp.2024.100304

[4] Oscar TP. Construction and validation of tertiary models for predicting growth of *Salmonella* Infantis in chicken liver during a processing chain deviation. Frontiers in Sustainable Food Systems. 2025;**9**:1565247. DOI: 10.3389/fsufs.2025.1565247

[5] Oscar TP. Poultry food assess risk model for *Salmonella* and chicken gizzards: III. Dose consumed step. Journal of Food Protection. 2024;**87**(4):100242. DOI: 10.1016/j.jfp.2024.100242

[6] Oscar TP. Poultry food assess risk model for *Salmonella* and chicken gizzards: II. Illness dose step. Journal of Food Protection. 2023;**86**(6):100091. DOI: 10.1016/j.jfp.2023.100091

[7] Oscar TP. Validation software tool (ValT) for predictive microbiology based on the acceptable prediction zones method. International Journal of Food Science and Technology. 2020;**55**(7):2802-2812. DOI: 10.1111/ijfs.14534

[8] Oscar TP. Poultry food assess risk model for *Salmonella* and chicken gizzards: I. Initial contamination. Journal of Food Protection. 2023;**86**(2):100036. DOI: 10.1016/j.jfp.2022.100036

[9] Thomas CJ, McMeekin TA. Attachment of *Salmonella* spp. to chicken muscle surfaces. Applied and Environmental Microbiology. 1981;**42**(1):130-134. DOI: 10.1128/aem.42.1.130-134.1981

[10] Thomas CJ, McMeekin TA. Contamination of broiler carcass skin during commercial processing procedures: An electron microscopic study. Applied and Environmental Microbiology. 1980;**40**(1):133-144. DOI: 10.1128/aem.40.1.133-144.1980

[11] Lillard HS. Comparison of sampling methods and implications for bacterial decontamination of poultry carcasses by rinsing. Journal of Food Protection. 1988;**51**(5):405-408. DOI: 10.4315/0362-028X-51.5.405

[12] Simmons M, Fletcher DL, Berrang ME, Cason JA. Comparison of sampling methods for the detection of *Salmonella* on whole broiler carcasses purchased from retail outlets. Journal of Food Protection. 2003;**66**(10):1768-1770. DOI: 10.4315/0362-028x-66.10.1768

[13] Parveen S, Taabodi M, Schwarz JG, Oscar TP, Harter-Dennis J, White DG. Prevalence and antimicrobial resistance of *Salmonella* recovered from processed poultry. Journal of Food

Protection. 2007;**70**(11):2466-2472. DOI: 10.4315/0362-028x-70.11.2466

[14] Surkiewicz BF, Johnston RW, Moran AB, Krumm GW. A bacteriological survey of chicken eviscerating plants. Food Technology. 1969;**23**(August):80-85

[15] Bemrah N, Bergis H, Colmin C, Beaufort A, Millemann Y, Dufour B, et al. Quantitative risk assessment of human salmonellosis from the consumption of a Turkey product in collective catering establishments. International Journal of Food Microbiology. 2003;**80**(1):17-30. DOI: 10.1016/s0168-1605(02)00145-9

[16] Oscar TP. Risk of salmonellosis from chicken parts prepared from whole chickens sold in flow pack wrappers and subjected to temperature abuse. Journal of Food Protection. 2017;**80**(9):1496-1505. DOI: 10.4315/0362-028X.JFP-17-097

[17] De Man JC. MPN tables, corrected. European Journal of Applied Microbiology and Biotechnology. 1983;**17**:301-305

[18] WHO FAO. Risk Assessments of *Salmonella* in Eggs and Broiler Chickens. Microbiological Risk Assessment Series 1. Geneva, Switzerland: World Health Organization and Food and Agricultural Organization; 2002. p. 34

[19] Oscar TP. Dose-response model for 13 strains of *Salmonella*. Risk Analysis. 2004;**24**(1):41-49. DOI: 10.1111/j.0272-4332.2004.00410.x

[20] Oscar TP. A quantitative risk assessment model for *Salmonella* and whole chickens. International Journal of Food Microbiology. 2004;**93**(2):231-247. DOI: 10.1016/j.ijfoodmicro.2003.12.002

[21] Smadi H, Sargeant JM. Quantitative risk assessment of human salmonellosis in Canadian broiler chicken breast from retail to consumption. Risk Analysis. 2013;**33**(2):232-248. DOI: 10.1111/j.1539-6924.2012.01841.x

[22] Juneja VK, Valenzuela Melendres M, Huang L, Gumudavelli V, Subbiah J, Thippareddi H. Modeling the effect of temperature on growth of *Salmonella* in chicken. Food Microbiology. 2007;**24**(4):328-335. DOI: 10.1016/j.fm.2006.08.004

[23] Oscar TP. General regression neural network and Monte Carlo simulation model for survival and growth of *Salmonella* on raw chicken skin as a function of serotype, temperature, and time for use in risk assessment. Journal of Food Protection. 2009;**72**(10):2078-2087. DOI: 10.4315/0362-028x-72.10.2078

[24] Murphy RY, Duncan LK, Johnson ER, Davis MD, Smith JN. Thermal inactivation D- and z-values of *Salmonella* serotypes and *Listeria innocua* in chicken patties, chicken tenders, franks, beef patties, and blended beef and Turkey patties. Journal of Food Protection. 2002;**65**(1):53-60. DOI: 10.4315/0362-028x-65.1.53

[25] Stathas L, Aspridou Z, Koutsoumanis K. Quantitative microbial risk assessment of *Salmonella* in fresh chicken patties. Food Research International. 2024;**178**:113960. DOI: 10.1016/j.foodres.2024.113960

[26] Oscar TP. Modeling the effect of inoculum size on the thermal inactivation of *Salmonella* Typhimurium to elimination in ground chicken thigh meat. American Journal of Food Science and Technology. 2017;**5**(4):135-142. DOI: 10.12691/ajfst-5-4-3

[27] Ross T. Indices for performance evaluation of predictive models in food microbiology. Journal of Applied

Bacteriology. 1996;**81**(5):501-508. DOI: 10.1111/j.1365-2672.1996.tb03539.x

[28] Halaji M, Heiat M, Faraji N, Ranjbar R. Epidemiology of COVID-19: An updated review. Journal of Research in Medical Sciences: The Official Journal of Isfahan University of Medical Sciences. 2021;**26**:82. DOI: 10.4103/jrms.JRMS_506_20

[29] McCullough NB, Eisele CW. Experimental human salmonellosis: II. Immunity studies following experimental illness with *Salmonella meleagridis* and *Salmonella anatum*. Journal of Immunology. 1951;**66**(5):595-608

[30] Araf Y, Akter F, Tang YD, Fatemi R, Parvez MSA, Zheng C, et al. Omicron variant of SARS-CoV-2: Genomics, transmissibility, and responses to current COVID-19 vaccines. Journal of Medical Virology. 2022;**94**(5):1825-1832. DOI: 10.1002/jmv.27588

[31] CDC. COVID Data Tracker. 2023 August 29. 2023. Available from: https://covid.cdc.gov/covid-data-tracker/#datatracker-home

[32] Anonymous. National Enteric Disease Surveillance: *Salmonella* Annual Report, 2016. 2018. Available from: https://www.cdc.gov/nationalsurveillance/pdfs/2016-Salmonella-report-508.pdf

Chapter 10

Perspective Chapter: One Health Approach Impact in *Salmonella* Public Health – Nexus with Molecular Mechanisms of Antimicrobial Resistance

Imad Mohamedtahir Fadlalla

Abstract

Salmonellosis encompasses a broad category of diseases, which may manifest as acute gastroenteritis, bacteremia, and extra intestinally localized infections affecting many organs in humans and animals. *Salmonella* strains that are multidrug-resistant have been one of the biggest global public health issues. Antibiotic-resistant bacteria are becoming more common, which may be related to the improper or unregulated use of antibiotics in animal experiments. A global public health concern is the rise in drug resistance in both humans and animals to commonly used antimicrobial medicines. Bacterial cells are multicellular populations that are well organized and able to integrate information from both their surroundings and themselves. It is clear that the global spread of antimicrobial-resistant mutants is a much more complicated event than can be achieved by using a vast number of individual cells. The idea that bacteria are solitary entities is not a realistic representation of the microbial world in nature. We should not just search for molecular cues that can affect the generation of antimicrobial-resistant mutants in order to obtain a comprehensive picture of bacterial antimicrobial resistance. We should keep in mind that physical fields are another way that bacterial cells can interact. Even though it is well established and scientifically significant that bacterial cells may produce sound and electromagnetic waves, this bacterial cell's potential is consistently disregarded. Although we can anticipate that molecular signals can contribute to the antimicrobial resistance alone, it is also possible to assume that multicellularity, outer membrane vesicles (OMVs), and physical signals can do.

Keywords: *Salmonella*, one health, public health, antimicrobial resistance, molecular mechanisms

1. Introduction

One of the most significant zoonotic foodborne pathogens in the world is *Salmonella*. Globally, *Salmonella* is estimated to be responsible for 155,000 deaths and 93 million enteric infections annually [1]. A toddler and an elderly person died from *Salmonella enterica* (SE) infections in 18 European nations between 2016 and 2020 [2]. Human gastrointestinal tract infections caused by *Salmonella* can result in diarrhea and even death. The intricate pathways of transmission include water, animal reservoirs, and the environment. Animals that produce food, especially poultry and livestock, are thought to be the main sources of SE infection in people [1]. There are just two main species in the genus *Salmonella*: *S. enterica* and *S. bongori*. There are six subspecies of *Salmonella enterica*. Subspecies of *enterica*, *salamae, arizonae, diarizonae, houtenae,* and *indica* are among them. According to the Kauffmann-White scheme, *Salmonella* strains are categorized into serovars based on the wide variety of lipopolysaccharide (LPS) antigens (O) and flagellar protein antigens (H); at this time, there are approximately 2500 serovars identified (Afolami and Onifade [3]).

Salmonellae have been linked to a broad range of diseases, from gastroenteritis and bacteremia to the potentially fatal typhoid. Some serovars of *Salmonella* exhibit extraordinary host adaptation; for example, serovars *Typhi, Dublin,* and *Gallinarum* infect humans, cattle, and birds, respectively. *Salmonella* is a facultative intracellular pathogen that usually colonizes reptiles, birds, and mammals (Falkow [4]). *Salmonella* species are significant animal and human zoonotic pathogens. Human health is at risk from animal *Salmonella* infections, especially if the affected animals' food products are consumed by humans (Liebisch and Schwarz [5]). A persistent *Salmonella* infection can lead to cancer and irritable bowel syndrome by disrupting the mucosal barrier, causing host immunological diseases, and upsetting the microbial community's equilibrium (Alenazy [6]).

Because of the close proximity to food animals, companion animals, live wildlife markets, environmental pollution, and the consumption of infected animal-derived foods, human and animal populations are susceptible to the direct transmission of zoonotic pathogens. Cross-transmission of antimicrobial resistance (AMR) determinants along with the infection makes matters more complex. Furthermore, in this intricate, multifaceted situation, the environmental resistance gene pool "resistome" also plays significant functions. Because human antibiotics are more readily available and of higher quality, companion animal practitioners prefer them, which leads to a disastrous situation. Due to high rates of morbidity, death, lost man-days, hospital length of stay (LOS), direct medical expenses, and the social costs of infection, antimicrobial resistance (AMR) causes massive financial losses [7]. An estimated 700,000 deaths annually were ascribed to AMR alone, surpassing the number of deaths from tuberculosis (TB), acquired immunodeficiency syndrome (AIDS), and malaria combined [8].

2. Integrating one health approach in *Salmonella* public health

Salmonella must not be present in 25 g of pooled neck skin samples from broiler carcasses, turkey carcasses, and the majority of food kinds, according to the modified European Union (EU) Regulation 2073/2005 to regulate *Salmonella* in the food chain. According to this rule, feeds that are ready to eat must be free of *Salmonella* [8].

Sampling must occur at least once every 16 weeks according to regulations. In 2018, the World Health Organization (WHO) issued guidelines for *Salmonella* control that address the entire food chain. By educating customers and training food handlers on best practices for preventing *Salmonella* and other foodborne illnesses, these initiatives seek to improve *Salmonella* monitoring efforts by fortifying food safety regulations. Consumers may be exposed to potentially fatal foodborne diseases as a result of poor hygiene procedures throughout the food chain, from harvesting or slaughter to processing, storage, distribution, transportation, and preparation [9, 10]. *Salmonella* in foods can spread as a result of inadequate food handling cleanliness, according to the United States Food and Drug Administration (USFDA). Poor food handling procedures in restaurants are the source of about 75% of these occurrences [11]. The risk of food risks can be decreased by using food workers who are properly trained and knowledgeable about food safety. All training is done in a brief period and so does not result in change in proper food safety behavior [8].

2.1 One health approach for *Salmonella* public health

According to Stanaway et al. [12], non-typhoidal *Salmonella* (NTS) continues to be a leading cause of illness and mortality globally. *Salmonella* caused a total of 180 million illnesses and 298,496 deaths in 2010, according to the WHO's Foodborne Disease Burden Epidemiology Reference Group (FERG). After assessing the health effects of every *Salmonella* serotype, Kirk et al. [13] came to the conclusion that this one poses the biggest foodborne burden. A total of 8.76 million Disability-Adjusted Life Years (DALYs) from all sources of transmission and 6.43 million attributable to contaminated foods were found when data related to *S. enterica* from diarrheal infections and the invasive non-typhoidal *Salmonella* (iNTS), *Salmonella typhi,* and *Salmonella Paratyphi A* were combined. Additionally, salmonellosis is the leading cause of food-related mortality worldwide and the second leading cause of gastroenteritis, according to Simpson et al. [14].

Animals are the source of major foodborne diseases like *Salmonella*, which are common in farm settings, and enter food supply chains. Understanding the many routes by which foodborne pathogens spread as well as identifying and mitigating hazards at every link in the food supply chain can be facilitated by the One Health approach [15]. It is widely acknowledged that the primary cause of salmonellosis is consuming contaminated food. One example of the One Health idea is the presence of bacteria in reservoirs in humans, domestic animals, and the environment [16]. The concept of "one health" recognizes how human, animal, and environmental well-being are all intertwined. According to Zinsstag et al. [17], the One Health concept has shown a lot of promise in tackling today's public health issues, especially those pertaining to newly developing infectious and zoonotic diseases. The number of human cases of salmonellosis will significantly decline as a result of the adoption of *Salmonella* control measures in poultry farms. Domesticated animals can contract bacteria from wild species, such as insects, rodents, mammals, and birds [18]. Through a variety of horizontal transfers, zoonotic bacteria have successfully traversed species borders and adapted to new hosts. Humans can contract salmonellosis by eating the meat of wildlife, including birds, reptiles, and wild boars, or by coming into close contact with these creatures. Numerous wild bird species, such as raptors, seagulls, crows, sparrows, pigeons, and waterfowl, have also been reported to contain varying amounts of *Salmonella* germs [19]. Because they frequently migrate between their feeding grounds and roosting or breeding regions, seabirds are essential to the ecosystem's ability to support zoonotic germs. Furthermore, during their yearly migrations, seabirds, like other bird species, can efficiently transfer disease through fecal contamination [20].

2.2 One health and antimicrobial resistance

According to estimates from the World Health Organization (WHO), AMR directly contributes to more than 1.27 million fatalities each year. By 2050, AMR may overtake cancer as the major cause of death, accounting for 10 million deaths annually, if nothing is done [21].

WHO compiled a list of medically important antimicrobials (MIAs) and divided them into three groups: important antimicrobials (IAs), highly important antimicrobials (HIAs), and critically important antimicrobials (CIAs, highest priority CIAs, and high priority CIAs). Similarly, based on the antimicrobial class, use in treating animal diseases, and availability of substitute antimicrobial agents, the World Organization for Animal Health (OIE) assessed the relative importance of several types of veterinary antimicrobial agents (Bandyopadhyay and Samanta [22]).

2.3 Possible sources of antimicrobial resistance in *Salmonella*

Modern healthcare systems face a serious problem with antibacterial drug resistance, which jeopardizes our capacity to treat bacterial infections. Developing more potent treatment plans against resistant microorganisms is made possible by an understanding of the forms and processes of antibiotic resistance [23].

2.3.1 Vegetable production

Certain antibiotics are used to prevent bacterial infections in crops, decorative plants, and lucrative fruits and vegetables. Another source of antimicrobial residue for fruits and vegetables is the manure used in soils and greenhouses [24]. An indirect indicator of AMR determinants (*tet, pAmpC*) was found in the untreated irrigation water used to produce crops, fruits, and vegetables [22]. Plants are not typically thought of as hosts for human infections like *Salmonella*. The danger of disease spread during preharvest and harvest is increased by fieldworkers' poor hygiene, the usage of portable restrooms, and handwashing stations (Ehuwa, et al. [8]).

2.3.2 Food animals

Antimicrobials are employed in animals for a variety of reasons, including growth promotion, prophylaxis, metaphylaxis, and treatment. However, it is vital to optimize the use of critically important antimicrobials (CIAs) and limit their usage to emergency situations or unique pathogenic diseases. The use of preventive antibiotics should not be used to make up for poor biosecurity and subpar farm husbandry circumstances. Using antibiotics on both healthy and at-risk animals in the same herd to stop the infection from spreading is known as metaphylaxis (Bandyopadhyay and Samanta [22]). International organizations like the World Health Organization (WHO), Food and Agricultural Organization (FAO), and World Organization for Animal Health (OIE) consider the use of medically important antimicrobials (MIAs) in animals for growth promotion, prophylaxis, and even metaphylaxis to be inappropriate antimicrobial usage (IAMU) [9, 10].

2.3.3 Companion animals

As pet welfare became more and more of a priority in contemporary culture, wealthy families began to treat their pets nearly like members of the family. The usage of antimicrobials and multidrug-resistant bugs has significantly expanded along with the rise in pet healthcare [25].

2.3.4 Aquaculture

Ponds and other open water aquaculture systems are heavily polluted by home and household activities, wastewater discharge, animal activity, and fertilizer with livestock manure (**Figure 1**). Since it is impractical to treat fish individually, antibiotics are administered en masse (metaphylactic) [26]. Due to inadequate intestinal absorption, fish often excrete the majority of antibiotics into the water and sediment, and waterbodies end up serving as antibiotic storage facilities, which puts selection pressure on the microflora (Bandyopadhyay and Samanta [22]). Humans can acquire antimicrobial resistance genes (ARGs) [27] through lateral transfer in the aquatic environment, thanks to transduction.

2.3.5 Household use of antimicrobials

Much emphasis was paid to the potential connection between the usage of disinfectants and the emergence of AMR. The possible link between the use of disinfectants triclosan in antibacterial soap and the development of AMR [28]. Sodium hypochlorite is frequently used in water chlorination, sewage cleanup, and household cleaning. It has been noted that chlorination increases resistance to ampicillin, ceftazidime, and chloramphenicol. It has been discovered that benzalkonium chloride (BAC), a quaternary ammonium used as a preservative in eye, ear, or nasal drops, can cause resistance even to antibiotics used as a last resort, such as polymyxin [29]. Other quaternary ammonium compounds have been reported to influence resistance to a variety of antimicrobials, including phenicol compounds, β-lactams, and quinolones, at subinhibitory doses (Bandyopadhyay and Samanta [22]).

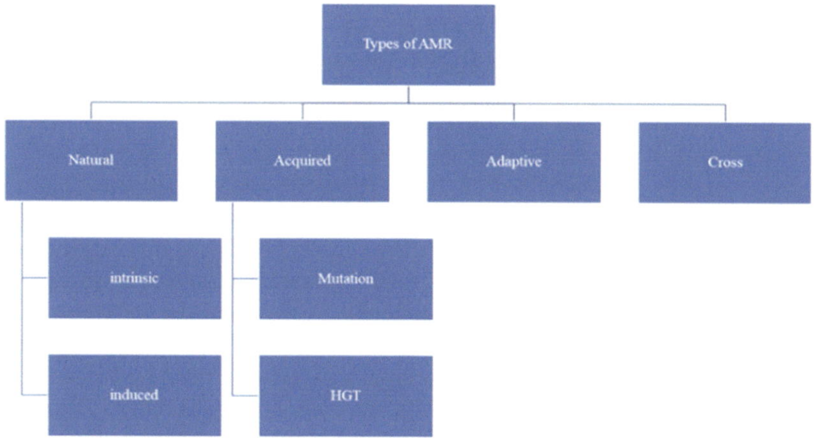

Figure 1.
Types of antimicrobial resistance.

2.4 One health approach for antimicrobial stewardship

One of the main causes of the development and spread of resistance in veterinary medicine continues to be the abuse and overuse of antimicrobials. Antimicrobials are commonly used in animals for growth promotion, disease prevention, and metaphylactic purposes, accounting for around 70% of all antibiotics supplied globally. The prevalence of over-the-counter antibiotics, inadequate regulatory supervision, and a lack of diagnostic tools all contribute to the danger of resistance in many nations [30]. Via food chains, direct contact, and environmental exposure, resistance genes in foodborne pathogens, such *Salmonella* spp., are progressively being passed from cattle to people. AMR mitigation can be approached holistically with the One Health framework, which acknowledges the connection of environmental, animal, and human health [31]. To decrease the use of antibiotics while maintaining food security and animal health, this approach prioritizes cross-sectoral cooperation, evidence-based recommendations, and surveillance systems [32]. In order to ensure adherence to global best practices, veterinarians are essential in educating farmers, keeping an eye on antibiotic use, and putting antimicrobial stewardship policies into place [33]. The prevalence of inferior or fake antibiotics, which increase the risk of resistance, uncontrolled antibiotic sales, and restricted access to diagnostics are some of the major obstacles that low- and middle-income countries (LMICs) must overcome. In human, animal, and environmental microbiomes, commensal bacterial strains function as silent repositories of genes causing antibiotic resistance, in addition to pathogenic bacteria. Despite not being harmful, these bacteria carry and spread resistance genes by conjugation, transformation, and transduction, three horizontal gene transfer methods. Multidrug-resistant (MDR) bacteria are commonly found in the gut microbiota of livestock and wildlife, and they can subsequently spread to bacterial communities linked to humans [34].

By 2050, 10 million fatalities could be attributed to antimicrobial resistance (AMR), according to a 2014 Review on AMR. One AMR was positioned as one of the twenty-first century's most urgent health dangers, thanks to this estimation. In accordance with the AMR Global Action Plan in 2016, a high-level United Nations (UN) General Assembly focused on AMR, and a Sustainable Development Goal (SDG) was added that specifically addressed AMR: lowering the proportion of bloodstream infections caused by particular antimicrobial-resistant organisms. A global assessment of the burden of bacterial AMR in 2019 was a significant advancement in AMR epidemiology, revealing that, of the approximately 8.9 million deaths resulting from bacterial infections that year, 1.27 million were directly related to AMR and 4.95 million were linked to AMR (Antimicrobial Resistance Collaborators [35]).

The One Health approach's main strategies for combating AMR are explained: 1. Raise awareness of the danger that comes from the overuse and abuse of antibiotics on a worldwide scale. 2. Strengthen and enhance hygienic practices to stop the spread of illnesses. 3. Cut down on the needless application of antibiotics in farming and the environmental contamination they cause. 4. Enhance medication resistance monitoring worldwide. 5. Encourage quick and innovative clinical diagnoses. 6. Encourage the creation and application of vaccinations and substitutes. 7. Acknowledge and expand the workforce that deals with infectious diseases. 8. Form an international alliance for effective AMR action [36].

Antimicrobial resistance may spread and circulate among people, animals, plants, and the environment in our globally interconnected world, making a "One Health" approach necessary. The WHO [37] states that there is an urgent need for new antibiotics to combat infections. *Salmonella*, which is fluoroquinolone-resistant (**Table 1**),

Priority	Pathogen list requiring new antimicrobials
Priority 1: Critical	• *Acinetobacter baumannii*: carbapenem-resistant
	• *Pseudomonas aeruginosa*: carbapenem-resistant
	• *Enterobacteriaceae*: carbapenem-resistant, ESBL-producing
Priority 2: High	• *Enterococcus faecium*: vancomycin-resistant
	• *Staphylococcus aureus*: methicillin-resistant, vancomycin-intermediate and resistant
	• *Helicobacter pylori*: clarithromycin-resistant
	• *Campylobacter* spp.: fluoroquinolone-resistant
	• *Salmonellae*: fluoroquinolone-resistant
	• *Neisseria gonorrhoeae*: cephalosporin-resistant, fluoroquinolone-resistant
Priority 3: Medium	• *Streptococcus pneumoniae*: penicillin-non-susceptible
	• *Haemophilus influenzae*: ampicillin-resistant
	• *Shigella* spp.: fluoroquinolone-resistant

Source: Refs. WHO [38], Alenazy [6].

Table 1.
A list of pathogenic bacteria for which new antimicrobials are urgently needed.

Antibacterial drugs	Mechanism of resistance
Quinolone and fluoroquinolone resistance	Mutations affecting the quinolone resistance-determining region (QRDR) in DNA gyrase (topoisomerase II and topoisomerase IV)
Linezolid, chloramphenicol, and clindamycin	Methylation of the 23S ribosomal RNA (rRNA) by an enzyme encoded by the *cfr* gene
Linezolid resistance	Mutations in genes encoding domain V of the 23S rRNA
Macrolide resistance	Methylation of 23S ribosomal RNA (rRNA) through the action of Erythromycin resistance methyltransferase (Erm)
Nitrofurantoin resistance	Mutations in the nitroreductase genes *nfsA* and *nfsB*, and mutations in the *ribE* gene
Resistance to glycopeptides in enterococci	Acquisition of a group of genes known as van gene clusters resulting in alteration of the terminal d-Alanine-d-Alanine moiety to d-Alanine-d-Lactate
Trimethoprim-sulfamethoxazole resistance in enterococci	The capacity of enterococci to utilize exogenous folinic acid
Aminoglycoside and fluoroquinolone resistance	Mutations leading to the inactivation or downregulation of porin proteins, such as OprD, result in reduced permeability
Tetracycline resistance	Activation of the *tet* system (increased efflux)
β-lactam antibacterial resistance	Production of β-lactamases
Chloramphenicol resistance	Acetylation by chloramphenicol acetyltransferase
Aminoglycoside resistance	Modification of the structure of aminoglycosides by aminoglycoside-modifying enzymes (AMEs)

Source: Ref. Belay et al. [23].

Table 2.
Examples of antibacterial drug resistance mechanisms.

is one of the infections that requires the most attention. Antibiotics may not be able to control bacterial infections in the post-antibiotic period due to the emergence of multidrug (MDR) and extensive drug resistance (XDR) that eventually leads to pan drug resistance (PDR) **Table 2** (Alenazy [6]).

3. Types of antibacterial drug resistance

Three types of antimicrobial resistance can be distinguished: acquired resistance, adaptive resistance, and intrinsic resistance [39]. However, it seems appropriate to classify drug resistance as acquired, adaptive, and natural.

3.1 Natural resistance

There are two types of natural resistance: induced (where genes naturally present in the bacterium are only expressed to resistant levels following antibacterial exposure) and intrinsic (always present in the species). A bacterial species' intrinsic resistance is shared within itself, unrelated to horizontal gene transfer, and unaffected by previous exposure to antibiotics [40]. Antibacterial resistance is a result of restriction of antibacterial entry brought on by porin proteins. Gram-negative bacteria are resistant to vancomycin because their outer membranes are impermeable to big glycopeptides, which is an example of natural antibacterial resistance [23].

3.2 Acquired resistance

When a bacterium that was previously susceptible to an antibiotic acquires resistance, it can be due to a mutation or the acquisition of new genetic material from an outside source by horizontal gene transfer (HGT) [40]. It results from alterations, including mutations, in the chromosome's structure or extrachromosomal components, such as transposons or plasmids [23]. Mutations in the bacterial chromosome that occur spontaneously are the source of chromosomal resistance. Numerous physical (such as ultraviolet (UV) light) and chemical stimuli can cause these mutations, which alter the structure of bacterial cells. This may lead to changes in drug targets inside the cell or decreased permeability to medicines. Extrachromosomal genetic elements are necessary for extrachromosomal resistance and can be transmitted by integrons, transposons, and plasmids (Yuce [41]).

3.3 Adaptive drug resistance

Adaptive drug resistance refers to the ability of microbes to reversibly adapt and develop resistance to one or more antibacterials in reaction to particular environmental cues. The reaction of drug resistance to several environmental factors, including stress, growth phase, pH, ion concentrations, nutrition availability, or exposure to subinhibitory doses of antibacterials, is observed. Adaptive drug resistance is inherently transient [42, 43].

3.4 Cross-resistance

Some microbes that exhibit resistance to one drug may also exhibit resistance to other medications that function similarly. The resistance between cephalosporins and penicillins is one example of how this phenomenon is frequently encountered in antibacterials with similar structures. Cross-resistance, however, can occasionally arise between pharmacological classes that are wholly unrelated. The cross-resistance between erythromycin and lincomycin serves as an illustration of this [44].

3.5 Multidrug resistance and pan-drug resistance

There are two primary ways that bacteria might become multidrug-resistant (MDR). First, bacteria can develop several genes, frequently carried on resistance (R) plasmids, each of which confers resistance to a particular antibiotic. Second, enzymatic inactivation, changes in target structure, elevated expression of genes encoding multidrug efflux pumps, and other processes can result in MDR. Multidrug-resistant bacterial strains are those that are resistant to three or more antimicrobial classes. Strains are categorized as widely drug-resistant if they exhibit resistance to all but one or two antibacterial classes [23]. According to Manchanda et al. [45], strains that are resistant to all available antibacterials are referred to be pan-drug-resistant.

4. Molecular mechanisms of *Salmonella* antimicrobial resistance

A variety of antibiotics, such as ampicillin, amoxicillin, gentamicin, trimethoprim/sulfamethoxazole, and fluoroquinolones, can be used to treat human salmonellosis. Numerous isolates exhibit resistance to at least one antibiotic [46]. Antibiotic resistance in *Salmonella* species is typically caused by both extended hospital stays and inadequate prophylactic antibiotic usage. Penicillin, aminoglycosides, tetracycline, cephalosporin, macrolides, ketolides, and several other antibiotics are among those to which the *Salmonella* spp had developed resistance against.

The suboptimal use of antibiotics for infection prevention and treatment, noncompliance with infection-control procedures, extended hospital stays, longer stays in intensive care units, multiple comorbidities in hospitalized patients, increased use of invasive devices and catheters, ineffective infection-control procedures, transfer of colonized patients from one hospital to another, placement of colonized patients in long-term-care facilities, and increased domestic and international travel are all contributing factors to the rise in antibiotic resistance levels in many *Salmonella* isolates [3].

4.1 Biochemical mechanisms of antimicrobial drug resistance

Generally, pathogenic bacteria have defenses against a variety of threats, the most significant of which being antibiotics. Among these methods are (i) efflux pumps, which extract the medications from bacterial cells and release them to the external environment, reducing their potency to non-toxic levels. (ii) Bacterial enzymes that alter or break down the structure of antibiotics inactivate them. (iii) Target site alteration through spontaneous mutation, which typically takes place in the cell envelope by changing the molecular targets' chemical structure. (vi) Blocking medication entry by altering the bacterial envelope's porin channels' frequency, size, and selectivity [47].

Bacteria can become resistant to antibacterials through four main mechanisms. These include changes to the antibacterials' target site, structural or enzymatic breakdown of antibacterials, the use of efflux pumps to maintain intracellular antibacterial concentrations below inhibitory levels, and modifications to the cell membrane's permeability [48].

Mechanisms, such as drug target change, drug inactivation, and drug efflux, are frequently involved in acquired resistance in bacteria. On the other hand, restricting drug uptake, drug inactivation, and drug efflux are the primary causes of intrinsic resistance [49]. All four of the main drug resistance pathways have been found to be used by Gram-negative bacteria [50].

4.1.1 Modification (alteration) of the drug target

One of the primary processes by which bacteria limit the efficacy of antibacterials is by mutating, modifying, or shielding their cellular targets, so disrupting the binding of the antibacterials [51]. Bacteria can become less susceptible to antibacterial medications by altering the shape of their cell wall, membrane, or other biological components that are targeted by these medications [52].

4.1.1.1 Target site alteration (by mutation or enzymatic alteration)

The targets required for drug binding can be changed by bacteria, which stop the drug from binding to the modified target at all or only partially. These changes frequently result from unplanned mutations in the gene or genes that code for the protein that the medication is intended to target. For instance, both Gram-positive and Gram-negative bacteria develop quinolone and fluoroquinolone resistance as a result of mutations that impact the quinolone resistance-determining region (QRDR) in DNA gyrase (topoisomerase II and topoisomerase IV) [53]. Target site change occurs when antibiotics' intended targets undergo alterations that prevent the medications from binding correctly, rendering them ineffective. The 23S ribosomal RNA (rRNA) genes are normally found in several copies in bacteria, and an increase in the number of mutant alleles is correlated with a higher minimum inhibitory concentration (MIC). Cross-resistance to macrolides, lincosamides, and streptogramin B (MLSB) results from the methylation of the 23S rRNA by enzymes that are encoded by different erm (erythromycin ribosome methylase) genes. The MLSB phenotype is the name given to this phenomenon [54].

4.1.1.2 Target replacement or target bypass

As an antibiotic resistance mechanism, target bypass or target substitution occurs when bacteria create alternative routes or substitute molecules that perform the same function as the original target. The development of van gene clusters, a collection of genes, results in resistance to glycopeptides. These genes reduce the binding affinity of the antibacterial molecule by facilitating the substitution of the glycopeptide target, specifically the terminal d-Alanine-d-Alanine moiety of peptidoglycan precursors. Due to the acquisition of the *vanA* gene cluster from vancomycin-resistant enterococci, there have been documented cases of high-level vancomycin resistance [23].

Transferable resistance to these antimicrobial agents has been linked to the acquisition of *dihydrofolate reductase* (DHFR) and *dihydropteroate synthase* (DHPS) genes, which encode enzymes resistant to trimethoprim and sulfonamide, respectively. Sometimes cells create resistance by adding a step that deviates from their normal physiological process. This usually requires another enzyme to be present. For example, trimethoprim resistance is conferred in *Escherichia coli* and *Citrobacter* sp. by the synthesis of an additional dihydrofolate reductase, which is identified by an R-plasmid. Furthermore, the antibacterial target may be produced in large quantities, effectively overwhelming the antibacterial, leading to resistance [55].

4.1.1.3 Target site protection

A molecule that mimics the antibacterial target can be produced by bacteria, which binds to the antibacterial and lowers its effective concentration. The *MfpA* protein, which is made up of pentapeptide repeats that resemble the charge and shape of B-DNA, is one example. By binding to DNA gyrase, the quinolone target, *MfpA* reduces the amount of *gyrase* available for quinolone binding, hence conferring resistance to quinolones. Furthermore, both Gram-positive and Gram-negative bacteria have been found to contain ribosomal protection proteins (RPPs), which work as an example of AMR through target site protection [23].

4.1.2 Decreased entry (influx) of antibacterials

Porins in the outer membrane are the primary means by which antibacterials enter the cell [51]. A bacterial cell's ability to enter antibacterials can be hindered by changes in the permeability of the outer membrane. This stops it from getting to the part of the bacteria that the antibiotic is trying to reach. Porin channels found in the outer membrane of Gram-negative bacteria have a significant impact on their ability to absorb antibacterials. Reduced permeability to different antibiotic classes, such as aminoglycosides and fluoroquinolones, is the consequence of mutations that cause porin proteins, including *OprD*, to become inactive or downregulated [56]. Lipid-rich outer membrane facilitates hydrophobic medications to enter the cell. However, the availability of hydrophilic medications is restricted by this hydrophobic barrier [57].

Hydrophilic antibacterials (such β-lactams, fluoroquinolones, tetracyclines, and chloramphenicol) enter bacteria mostly through porins in the outer membrane. According to Fernández and Hancock [58] and Choi and Lee [59], the number and type of porins expressed on the outer membrane affect the penetration of hydrophilic antibacterials and, in turn, the bacterial cell's susceptibility to these antibacterials. Porin mutations can take many different forms, such as decreased expression of the porin, changes in its size or conductance, or deletion of the porin.

4.1.3 Increased expression of efflux pumps

Efflux pumps are complicated bacterial mechanisms that rely on energy and are found on the cytoplasmic membrane. They are able to remove harmful molecules, such as drugs, from the cell, which lower the drug's concentration and reduce its potency. By removing antibacterials from bacterial cells, they lower the intracellular concentration and effectiveness of these drugs, which greatly contribute to multidrug resistance [47]. The efficiency of antibacterial medications may be diminished by mutations that result in the overexpression of efflux pumps, which lowers the concentration of antibacterials at the target site. The bacterial chromosome is primarily responsible for encoding multidrug efflux systems. Mobile genetic elements frequently contain genes encoding substrate-specific efflux pumps [58]. Examples of substrate-specific efflux pumps are those designed for macrolides, chloramphenicol, and tetracyclines [49].

Primary and secondary transporters are the two types of bacterial transport proteins that make up efflux pumps, which remove toxins and medications from bacterial cells [6]. Adenosine triphosphate (ATP) binding and hydrolysis activate primary transporters, which are members of the ATP-binding cassette (ABC) family and aid efflux. Conversely, secondary transporters include a number of families, including the drug metabolite transporter (DMT) superfamily, the resistance nodulation division (RND) family, the small multidrug resistance (SMR) family, the multidrug and toxic compound extrusion (MATE) family, and the major facilitator superfamily (MFS) [60]. In Gram-negative bacteria, the RND superfamily usually contains the main clinically significant efflux mechanisms. These systems typically include a cytoplasmic membrane pump, a periplasmic protein, and an outer-membrane protein channel [61]. This resistance decreases the bacterium's susceptibility to fluoroquinolones, tetracycline, tigecycline, chloramphenicol, erythromycin, trimethoprim, netilmicin, and meropenem [62]. RND pump overactivity leads to quinolone resistance. One of the main pumps causing efflux-mediated resistance is the *tet* system [63]. It uses a proton exchange mechanism to remove tetracycline.

4.1.4 Enhanced secretion of antibacterial inactivating (modifying) enzymes

The ability of a bacterium to create enzymes that either degrade or change antibacterials, making them useless, is a therapeutically significant resistance mechanism. *β-Lactamases*, *aminoglycoside-modifying enzymes*, and *chloramphenicol acetyltransferases* are the three primary enzymes that deactivate antibacterials [49]. When some bacterial species inactivate antibacterials, either by transferring a chemical group to the antibacterial or by degrading the antibacterial, drug resistance may result [51]. Hydrolysis can easily change the hydroxyl and amide groups in an antibacterial's structure. Furthermore, antibacterials can be rendered inactive by adding acetyl, phosphate, and nucleotide groups [64].

4.1.4.1 β-Lactamases

Both chromosomes and mobile genetic elements (MGEs) can include genes that encode β-lactamases. TEM-1 is a β-lactamase that is encoded by a plasmid. Third-generation cephalosporins can be hydrolyzed by plasmid-encoded β-lactamases called Extended-Spectrum β-*Lactamases* (ESBLs). Serine β-lactamases with active sites fall under class A. Metallo-β-lactamases that depend on a divalent metal ion, usually Zn2+, for their activity are classified as class B. Class C or *AmpC β-lactamases* and class D *β-lactamases* are classified as well [23]. A wide range of β-lactam antibiotics with ester and amide linkages can be hydrolyzed by β-lactamases. Among these include carbapenems, monobactams, cephalosporins, and penicillins [65]. Gram-negative bacteria have a subclass of class A β-lactamases called ESBLs. β-Lactamase inhibitors block cephamycins and carbapenems, but they confer resistance to penicillins, first-, second-, and third-generation cephalosporins, and aztreonam. According to Tamma et al. [66], ESBLs can also provide resistance to non-β-lactam drugs, such as aminoglycosides, trimethoprim-sulfamethoxazole, nitrofurantoin, and fluoroquinolones. Additionally, AmpC, a subtype of class C β-lactamase enzymes, confers resistance to cephamycins, aztreonam, penicillins, and first-, second-, and third-generation cephalosporins, but not carbapenems. Furthermore, a wide range of enzymes, known as carbapenemases, provide resistance to carbapenems; many of these enzymes also give resistance to nearly all hydrolyzable β-lactams [67]. Furthermore, some *Enterobacteriaceae* are capable of producing carbapenemase enzymes, which make cephalosporins, penicillins, and carbapenems ineffective [68].

4.1.4.2 Aminoglycoside inactivating enzymes

By altering the structure of aminoglycoside molecules, aminoglycoside-modifying enzymes (AMEs) reduce their affinity and prevent them from binding to the 30S ribosomal subunit. According to Strateva and Yordanov [69], AMEs provide broad-spectrum resistance to fluoroquinolones (FQs) and aminoglycosides (AGs). AMEs help modify antibacterials with a lower affinity for their target by facilitating aminoglycoside acetylation, phosphorylation, or adenylation [70].

4.1.4.3 Acetylation

Acetylation is often used as a defense mechanism against fluoroquinolones, streptogramins, and chloramphenicol [49]. *Chloramphenicol acetyltransferase* is an enzyme produced by Gram-negative bacteria that acetylates the hydroxyl groups of chloramphenicol. This modified chloramphenicol loses its ability to attach to the 50S ribosomal subunit correctly due to acetylation **Figure 2** [23].

4.2 Outer membrane vesicles (OMVs)

Microorganisms must communicate with their surroundings in order to survive and adapt within a host. In every domain, the release of extracellular vesicles (EVs) and cellular chemicals into the environment is essential for interactions between and within species [71]. Both Gram-positive and Gram-negative bacterial species have been examined for their ability to secrete membrane vesicles (MVs). Gram-positive bacteria refer to these vesicles as cytoplasmic membrane vesicles (CMVs), whereas

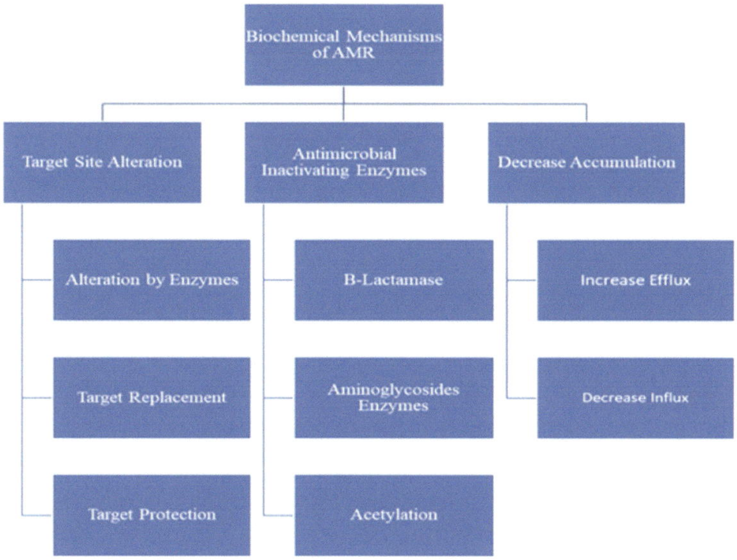

Figure 2.
The biochemical mechanisms of antimicrobial resistance (AMR).

Gram-negative bacteria call them outer membrane vesicles (OMVs) [72]. During Gram-negative bacterial phase growth, OMVs—small, spherical, bilayered structures with dimensions ranging from 20 to 350 nm—are released [73].

Antibiotic treatment causes stress responses in susceptible bacteria, which result in the release of OMVs. In order to counteract the effects of antibiotics and other antimicrobial substances, OMVs might be crucial. By serving as physical barriers that bind and absorb antimicrobial peptides or phages, decoys prevent bacteria from being eradicated [74]. Additionally, it has been noted that bacterial strains that are resistant to antibiotics release OMVs that contain β-lactamase, which reduces the efficiency of β-lactam antibiotics against these strains [75]. The ability of OMVs to impact other antibiotics, including polymyxin B, melittin, and colistin, has been discovered. A new function of OMVs that is closely linked to antimicrobial resistance (AMR) has also been discovered by another research. The transfer of antimicrobial resistance genes (ARGs) across bacteria is the foundation of this mechanism. Horizontal gene transfer is how genetic material, including ARGs, is packaged into OMVs and transferred. This makes it easier for OMV to spread drug-resistant genes throughout microbial populations, which in turn make it possible for bacteria to pick up resistance genes from even distant relatives [73].

A wide range of physiological processes, such as quorum sensing, horizontal gene transfer, intracellular and extracellular communication, interbacterial killing, toxin transport, polysaccharide hydrolysis, and stress responses, have been linked to OMVs (**Figure 3**) [76].

4.2.1 Bacterial EVs bind or encapsulate antibiotics

A phospholipid bilayer makes up the majority of the bacterial cell membrane. This membrane structure regulates the inflow and outflow of chemicals, in addition to acting as a barrier to protect germs [77]. Daptomycin and polymyxin B, for example, are membrane-targeting antibiotics that can attach to phospholipids or

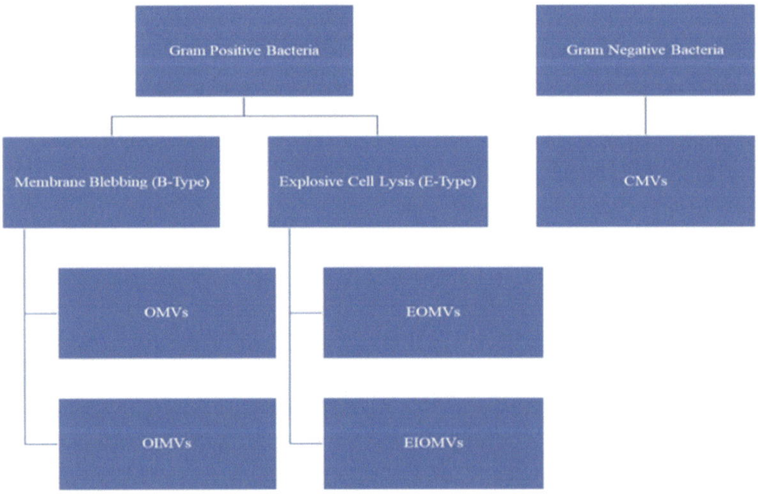

Figure 3.
Types and biogenesis of bacterial EVs. Outer membrane vesicles (OMVs), Outer-inner membrane vesicles (OIMVs), Explosive-inner outer membrane vesicles (EIOMVs), Explosive-outer membrane vesicles (EOMVs), and Cytoplasmic membrane vesicles (CMVs).

lipopolysaccharides (LPSs) on the bacterial cell membrane, respectively. This compromises the integrity of the membrane and kills the bacteria. It is clear that OMVs and CMVs can both serve as decoys to attach to antibiotics that target membranes and offer protection. Furthermore, bacteria will release antibiotic-carrying EVs when they are exposed to antibiotics. This implies that antibiotics were included within the EVs. Because efflux pumps are highly expressed in bacteria, antibiotics are expelled from the cell as OMVs. Membrane bending may result from antibiotics that interact with bacterial LPS, such as gentamicin. Antibiotics may be encapsulated in OMVs as a result of this. Furthermore, endolysin expression can be activated by antibiotics that break DNA, such as ciprofloxacin, which can cause explosive cell lysis [76]. Antibiotics may therefore be encapsulated by explosive outer-inner membrane vesicles (EOIMVs) and explosive outer membrane vesicles (EOMVs) while they are being assembled.

4.2.2 Bacterial EVs degrade antibiotics through antibiotic-degrading enzymes

β-Lactamases can be transported outside of cells by bacterial EVs [78]. This occurs because bacteria that produce β-lactamases can use the Sec system to move the enzymes to the periplasmic region when they are under antibiotic stress. The β-lactamases are then transferred outside of the cell after being encapsulated into EVs via advantageous electrostatic protein-membrane contacts [79]. To protect bacteria, these EVs that carry *β-lactamases* can break down nearby drugs. The porins on the surface of bacterial EVs are involved in degrading process. Proteins called porins create channels on the outer membrane of bacteria that let small molecules to enter. Antibiotics are thus hydrolyzed by internal *β-lactamases* after being absorbed by bacterial EVs through these porins. When porins are not present, EVs' capacity to degrade antibiotics is greatly reduced. Furthermore, by lowering antibiotic concentrations, bacterial EVs can encourage bacterial porin mutations [76].

4.2.3 Bacterial EVs transfer resistance genes to recipient cell

Through the transfer of resistance genes, EVs can also mediate the spread of resistance. Only OIMVs, EOMVs, EOIMVs, and CMVs have the potential to transport DNA, although classic OMVs usually do not. This is due to the fact that OMVs cannot contain cytoplasmic contents because their biogenesis method solely requires the bacterial outer membrane. When EVs carrying DNA come into touch with the outer membrane of the bacteria, they lyse it. Type IV pili then carry the DNA into the cytoplasm. This implies that the receivers' proficiency may have an impact on the uptake of EV-associated DNA [80].

Environmental factors including temperature, pH, stress levels, and nutrition availability also affect the composition of bacterial extracellular vesicles (BEVs), causing changes that maximize bacterial communication and survival. Furthermore, the selective packing of particular bioactive molecules is determined by the functional role of BEVs, which may include pathogenesis, intercellular communication, antibiotic resistance, or host immunological regulation [81]. Gram-negative bacteria have three membranes: an inner membrane (IM), a periplasmic space, and an outer membrane (OM). These membranes affect how BEVs form. Outer membrane vesicles (OMVs) and outer-inner membrane vesicles (OIMVs) are the two main vesicles that they release. Lipopolysaccharides (LPSs), outer membrane proteins, phospholipids, and periplasmic components are all present in OMVs, which are produced exclusively from the outer membrane [72]. Because OIMVs include both inner and outside membrane components, cytoplasmic proteins and nucleic acids can be packaged [82].

4.2.4 Role of BEVs in antibiotic resistance

By a variety of methods, BEVs contribute to the development of antibiotic resistance in bacterial populations. The first function of BEVs is to facilitate horizontal gene transfer by enclosing and spreading resistance genes throughout bacterial cells, even between species. BEVs can also cause antibiotic resistance through the breakdown or sequestration of drugs. Additionally, exposure to antibiotics frequently raises the production of BEV. By exporting toxic compounds from the cell or neutralizing antibiotics, these vesicles can shield vulnerable bacteria within a population. Thirdly, by hindering antibiotic penetration, BEVs aid in the production of biofilms, a crucial resistance strategy [82].

4.3 Multicellularity

4.3.1 Transient hypermutators

When a single mutation was needed to solve a specific problem, the adaptive mutants emerged. An adaptive mutation process may be the cause of solutions requiring many mutations at once, according to the most widely accepted "hypermutable state" model [83]. According to this "hypermutable state" paradigm, a tiny bacterial population experiences a brief period of high mutation rate during a protracted non-lethal selection process. A cell in this hypermutable condition starts to grow and procreate while simultaneously leaving the hypermutable state if it makes a beneficial mutation that relieves the selection pressure (Krašovec, and Jerman [84]).

The hypermutable model states that a bacterial culture has two populations when subjected to non-lethal antibiotic selection pressure. There is a primary population with normal mutational rates and a tiny population known as hypermutators with high mutational rates. Only antibiotic-resistant mutants that require mutations in many targets may be caused by transitory hypermutators. These genes can be actively transferred to nearby colonies by a hypermutator, resulting in the formation of normal cells. Natural competence, the physiological state that permits bacterial cells to transfer and integrate foreign resistance genes into the chromosome, is strikingly similar to the temporary hypermutable state [85]. The similarity is evident in the fact that both phenomena include a mechanism that keeps most of the population genetically stable while allowing a small portion of the population to become more genetically variable. Resistance genes may be released by hypermutators during autolysis or deliberately expelled into the environment, where they would be absorbed and integrated into the chromosome by other cells [86].

4.3.2 Bacterial biofilms

The majority of bacteria live in biofilms in nature. Dense collections of one or more bacterial species bound together by a hydrated matrix of proteins and polysaccharides are called biofilms. The ability of bacteria to communicate with one another is essential for the multicellular developmental process of biofilm formation (Krašovec and Jerman [84]).

Bacterial cells in a biofilm are likely to either not divide at all or divide very slowly when they are subjected to selective pressure from an antibiotic. This reasoning is supported by the following facts: first, bacterial cells typically live in near-starvation conditions in nature; and second, certain bacteria may enter a non-growing state due to altered chemical microenvironment within a biofilm, including a gradient in nutrient concentration, inhibitory waste products, and oxygen accessibility. An antibiotic is likely to enter the biofilm more slowly than it would enter cells that are free-floating. Consequently, non-lethal antibiotic doses may be administered to at least a portion of the cells in a biofilm. Therefore, cells that are either nondividing or slowly dividing under a non-lethal selection pressure are both essential requirements for the adaptive mutation. One crucial mechanism of the overall antibiotic resistance of biofilms is the adaptive mutation process, which includes transient hypermutators. Furthermore, a highly significant method of dispersing the resistance may be an intercellular genetic mutation between hypermutators and healthy cells [87].

Flagella are produced by most bacterial species. The most prominent feature of creatures harboring flagella is their motility in liquid media (swimming), which enables a directed response to environmental cues (Harshey and Toguchi [88]). Additionally, flagella are involved in swarming, which is a type of multicellular behavior in bacteria that involves spreading on plates. Flagella can also act as adhesion agents to abiotic and biological surfaces because of their extracellular position (Moens and Vanderleyden [89]). A single protein's components make up the flagellin filament. Two genes, *fliC* (the phase-1 flagellin) and *fliB* (the phase-2 flagella), encode the filament protein in *Salmonella typhimurium* (Romling and Rohde [90]).

Multicellular behavior in bacteria can occur in various forms and is synonymous with the formation of biofilms, which are defined as "matrix-enclosed bacterial populations adherent to each other and/or to surfaces or interfaces." In *S. typhimurium*, a multicellular morphotype, the red, dry, and rough (rdar) morphotype, has been described [91]. Thin, aggregative fibers (*agf*) were recognized as a component of the extracellular matrix responsible for parts of the rdar morphology on plates, the formation of large cell clusters in liquid culture, and adherence to abiotic surfaces. Hyperflagellation was reported to occur in cells expressing the rdar morphotype on plates (Romling and Rohde [90]).

Biofilms are important in medicine because they have been linked to the etiology of a number of bacterial infections that are difficult to treat with antibacterials. They accomplish this by lowering the drug's ability to enter bacterial cells and by serving as a physical barrier that keeps the medication from getting to its intended target [92]. According to reports, AMR in biofilm formations is caused by a variety of causes. The first explanation is that, while some antibacterials may still be able to pass through the biofilm polysaccharide matrix, there is little diffusion of antibacterials across it. The second pathway involves physiological alterations brought on by sluggish development rates and reactions to environmental stress or hunger, such as nutrition and oxygen deprivation. Phenotypic alterations in the cells that make up the biofilm are the cause of the third mechanism. Quorum sensing is the reason for the other. The expression of efflux pumps is the fifth explanation. Persister cells, which are tiny fractions of bacteria that show persistence by avoiding eradication when exposed to antimicrobials, are linked to the final mechanism causing AMR in biofilm [23]. Quorum sensing, which involves identifying extracellular autoinducers, is how biofilms naturally form. This enhanced resistance is linked to quorum sensing, efflux pump expression, and the decreased capacity of antibacterials to permeate into the biofilm matrix [93].

4.4 Antimicrobial resistance genes

Antimicrobial resistance is caused either by mutations in chromosomal genes (intrinsic resistance) or by acquisition of plasmid-mediated resistance determinants (extrinsic resistance). The intrinsic resistance is mainly due to selection pressure whereas extrinsic genes are acquired by horizontal transfer [49]. The recent trends in the development of antimicrobial resistance (AMR) among *S. Typhi* proposed that multidrug-resistant (MDR) enteric fever was decreasing and being replaced by enteric fever with fluoroquinolone-resistant strains [94]. Similarly, hospital-based genomic surveillance for enteric fever, using whole-genome sequencing (WGS) method, suggested that large number of isolates showed non-susceptibility to fluoroquinolones [95]. Genome characterization assessment for AMR and pan-genome of clinical isolates in endemic countries like India will assist in recognition of variations in resistance mechanism and epidemiology, leading to better selection of antimicrobial therapy and implementation of appropriate preventive measures (Amit [96]).

The WGS analysis revealed that all strains have mutations in the *gyrA, gyrB, parC,* and *parE* genes that confer fluoroquinolone resistance. *CatA1* genes for chloramphenicol resistance, *dfrA7, dfrA15, sul1,* and *sul2* for trimethoprim-sulfamethoxazole, and bla_{TEM}-*116*/bla_{TEM}-*1B* genes for amoxicillin were among the acquired resistance-determining mechanisms found. For ceftriaxone and cefixime, no resistance determinants were discovered. For ampicillin, co-trimoxazole, ciprofloxacin, ceftriaxone, and chloramphenicol, the genotypes and corresponding phenotypes were further connected. In *S. Typhi* isolates, a strong association between genotypes and phenotypes was found. According to the pan-genome study, accessory genes were mostly linked to disease and antibiotic resistance, while core genes were enriched in metabolic processes. According to Heap's law analysis, the pan-genome of *S. Typhi* seems to be closed (Bpan = 0.09). A reduced degree of genetic diversity among *S. Typhi* isolates was indicated by Simpson's diversity index of 0.51. All things considered, this work adds to the current understanding that WGS can assist in predicting resistance genotypes and their eventual link with symptoms, providing the opportunity to identify AMR determinants for prompt diagnosis and to prioritize the usage of antibiotics straight from sequence [96].

Amino acid substitutions in the quinolone resistance-determining region (QRDR) of the genes *gyrA* and *parC* are the most common mechanism among strains resistant to quinolones and/or fluoroquinolones. However, plasmid-mediated quinolone resistance (PMQR), which is linked to the genes *qnrA, qnrB, qnrC, qnrD,* and *qnrS,* is becoming more significant, though its detection frequency varies. Genes *sul1* and *sul2* are mostly linked to resistance to sulfonamides, whereas different *dhfr (dfr)* gene variations are linked to resistance to trimethoprim. When considering *Salmonella* spp. strains that have been isolated from food, β-lactamases that are encoded by bla_{TEM} genes are frequently linked to resistance to β-lactam antibiotics. Nevertheless, AmpC-positive and ESBL strains are also seen. Enzymatic inactivation is frequently the cause of resistance to aminoglycosides. Acetyltransferases (AACs), *adenylyltransferases* (ANTs), and *aminoglycoside phosphotransferases* (APHs) are the three different kinds of enzymes that change aminoglycosides. When *Salmonella* species are isolated from food, active efflux is most frequently linked to tetracycline resistance. The most commonly documented genetic determinants encoding efflux pumps are *tetA, tetB, tetC, tetD, tetE,* and *tetG.* Chloramphenicol efflux pumps, which are expressed by the genes *cmlA* and *floR,* can also mediate resistance to chloramphenicol, but their inactivation by *chloramphenicol acetyltrasferases* (CATs) is one of the most prevalent routes of resistance to this chemical. Because globalization of trade leads to the long-distance movement of goods, animals, and food products, which promotes the spread of resistant diseases worldwide, it is crucial to keep an eye on the resistance of *Salmonella* isolated from food [97].

4.5 Mobile genetic elements

The capture, accumulation, and spread of AMR genes among bacterial populations, as well as the evolution of bacterial genomes through conjugation, transduction, or transformation, are all facilitated by mobile genetic elements (MGEs), which include integrons, phages (~11–500 kb in length), transposons (Tns) (~5 kb in length), insertion sequences (ISs) (~2.5 kb in length), integrative and conjugative elements (ICEs), integrons, and genomic islands [98]. The evolution of NTS, including the acquisition of virulence and AMR genes, is also greatly influenced by the horizontal transfer of foreign genes mediated by MGE [99].

A key factor in the quick evolution and adaptation of bacteria is horizontal gene transfer (HGT). According to Tokuda and Shintani [100], bacteria undergo HGT by a variety of processes, such as transformation, transduction, and conjugation.

Protein capsids that contain nucleic acids (DNA or RNA) that may infect and replicate within bacteria or archaea make up bacteriophages, also known as phages. The exchange of phage DNA and the host genome during integration and excision within the host genome, as well as the co-excision of nearby bacterial genes, can lead to the horizontal gene transfer (HGT) of certain genes, suggesting that phages are essential for fostering microbial evolution [101]. The nucleic acid composition, shape, presence or absence of capsid protein and its structure, nucleotide sequence similarity, and host range are among the characteristics that are used to identify or classified phages [102].

4.5.1 Plasmids

Conjugation is one way that plasmids, which are circular or linear extrachromosomal replicons, can be transmitted. Notably, conjugation is a significant phenomenon for the quick evolution and adaptability of bacteria since different genes can circulate among them efficiently. The host phenotype of two distinct plasmids is the basis for the incompatibility (Inc) classification. The compatibility of two plasmids can be impacted by additional characteristics outside the replication system, such as the partition system, surface exclusion, and entrance exclusion systems (Tokuda and Shintani [100]).

4.5.2 Chromosomally integrated MGEs

ICEs, integrative mobilizable elements (IMEs), and cis-mobilizable elements (CIMEs) are among the chromosomally integrated MGEs (ciMGEs) that have been found [103]. According to Delavat et al. [104], ICEs are self-transmissible conjugative elements that are usually incorporated into the host chromosome. Conjugation, which entails the creation of a mating pair with a type IV secretion system between donor and recipient cells, is the first step in the transfer of ICEs. A single-stranded DNA molecule is then transferred from the donor cell to the recipient cell. IMEs are similar to ICEs; however, they are not capable of self-transport. IMEs lack the genes necessary for conjugation, therefore even though they can integrate into host chromosomes, they need other conjugative elements, like conjugative plasmids or ICEs, to mobilize and transfer to other bacterial cells. The *integrase* of an ICE or IME that they are attached to recognizes the recombination sites (attL and attR) on either side of CIMEs, despite the fact that they lack the genes necessary for conjugation or recombination Tokuda and Shintani [100]. These elements, like plasmids, can carry genes that encode virulence factors, metabolic traits, and ARGs, among other things [105].

4.5.3 Transposons

Genetic elements known as transposons move between replicons by transposase activity. Transposons can enter other cells after being integrated into plasmids or ICEs, despite the fact that they are not intercellularly transferable). The transposase enzyme, which catalyzes transposon transposition, is typically encoded by a gene found in transposons. Terminal inverted repeat sequences (TIRs) surround one or two transposase genes to form insertion sequences (ISs), which are minimum transposons [106]. Genes carried by certain transposons aid in the dissemination of ARGs and other characteristics. Through homologous recombination, many copies of the same IS element can encourage genomic rearrangements [100].

4.5.4 Integrons

Despite not being transposed or transferred like transposons or chromosomally integrated mobile genetic elements (ciMGEs), integrons are genetic elements that are important in the transmission of ARGs among bacteria. Every integron has a class 1 integron-integrase gene (intI1), a promoter (Pc) in the inner region of intI1, and a recombination site (attI) [107]. Gene cassettes, which are tiny DNA pieces containing ARGs or other functional genes, are inserted into the attI site. The gene cassettes' attI and attC sites are recognized by IntI1, which then catalyzes the site-specific recombination between the two sites, causing the cassette to insert into the integron structure. Integrons, which include numerous gene cassettes in a single structure, have the ability to quickly accumulate and spread different ARGs among bacterial populations. Based on variations in intI1 sequences, integrons are categorized into multiple groups [108]. According to Gillings [109], class 1 integrons play the most significant role in the dissemination of ARGs among bacteria.

4.5.5 Horizontal gene transfer (HGT)

4.5.5.1 Conjugation

One of the most significant HGT processes is conjugation. In order to facilitate the transmission of genetic material, this procedure requires direct physical contact between bacterial cells. A sex pilus is created during conjugation, which makes it easier for a plasmid to be transferred to the recipient bacteria. The bacterium can acquire multidrug resistance if several drug resistance genes on the plasmid are transferred to it in a single conjugation event. Transposons, which are now categorized as Integrative Conjugative Elements (ICEs) or Integrative Mobilizable Elements (IMEs), can be conjugated, as can conjugative or nonconjugative plasmids [23].

Genomic islands are also a part of ICEs and IMEs. When other mobile elements supply the necessary transfer genes (*tra* genes), a nonconjugative plasmid can transfer. For genetic material to be transferred between Gram-positive and Gram-negative bacteria, these *tra* genes are essential. The presence of transposon insertion elements on the plasmids frequently facilitates plasmid fusion. According to Brochet et al. [110], genomic plasticity is facilitated by mobile genetic components. The IME known as *Salmonella* genomic island 1 (SGI1), which is present in several *Salmonella* serovars, is an illustration of adaptability. Ampicillin, chloramphenicol, florfenicol, streptomycin, spectinomycin, sulfonamide, and tetracycline resistance genes were found in the SGI1 [111].

However, a number of epidemiological and molecular reasons limit conjugation. The ecology must first allow the strains to come into touch with one another. Second, the stresses need to be somewhat mobile, either on their own or as a result of outside factors. Third, plasmids from the same incompatibility group may not be able to enter the same cell due to plasmid incompatibility. Fourth, the cell's genetic makeup must facilitate the IME's integration, especially for IMEs. Lastly, if certain mobile genetic components are expelled from the cell, their maintenance systems may result in cell death [112].

4.5.5.2 Transformation

Through the process of DNA recombination known as transformation, a microorganism absorbs exogenous DNA pieces, or naked DNA, from its surroundings and incorporates them into its genetic composition to produce inheritable features [113]. There are multiple steps involved in transformation. Bacterial DNA is first liberated from bacterial cells, either actively at particular stages of the development cycle for some bacteria or passively after death and lysis. After being released, the DNA is absorbed by surrounding competent bacteria. The DNA must then get firmly integrated into the acceptor cell and resist the potentially damaging activity of nucleases within the bacterial cell. Lastly, expression of the integrated DNA occurs [23].

Certain uptake sequences, usually found in the inverted repeats of donor sequences, are necessary for effective DNA uptake in Gram-negative model organisms. After binding, the DNA rapidly develops a resistance to DNase and is subsequently absorbed (Sikorski et al. [114]). Depending on the species, competence is induced differently. Throughout the logarithmic growth phase, certain species that are naturally transformable maintain their competence. Others only acquire competence at the beginning of the stationary phase and are competent for short periods of time. Despite using comparable proteins, Gram-positive and Gram-negative bacteria have different DNA absorption methods due to differences in their cell wall structure. The creation, upkeep, and gene transfer of bacterial biofilms may be significantly influenced by transformation [23].

4.5.5.3 Transduction

A bacteriophage and an infected bacteria exchange genetic material through a process known as transduction, which is a bacteriophage-mediated transfer [49]. The bacteriophage first clings to the bacterium and introduces its genetic material, which could comprise DNA from the host bacteria as well as the virus. The foreign DNA must be stabilized inside the bacterial cell, either by integrating into the bacterial DNA or by producing an element that replicates on its own. The foreign DNA can guide the creation of new phage particles once it has stabilized. Bacterial plasmids and/or genomic DNA of different lengths can be passed from one bacterium to another using this method. Because bacteriophages are host specific, transduction usually takes place between closely related bacterial strains. Therefore, transduction is the process by which a drug-resistance gene is transferred from a resistant bacterium to a nonresistant bacterium via a vector (bacteriophage) [23].

5. Conclusions

The misuse and overuse of antimicrobials in veterinary medicine remain key contributors to the emergence and dissemination of resistance. It is clear that the global spread of antimicrobial-resistant mutants is a much more complicated event than can be achieved by using a vast number of individual cells. The idea that bacteria are solitary entities is not a realistic representation of the microbial world in nature. We should not just search for molecular cues that can affect the generation of antimicrobial-resistant mutants in order to obtain a comprehensive picture of bacterial antimicrobial resistance.

Acknowledgements

I acknowledge and am grateful for the support and assistance that my colleagues have given me.

Conflict of interest

The author declares no conflict of interest.

Author details

Imad Mohamedtahir Fadlalla
Department of Genetic Research, Imam Abdulrahman Bin Faisal University, Institute of Research and Medical Consultation, Saudi Arabia

*Address all correspondence to: imadmohamedtahir@hotmail.com

References

[1] Liu B, Zhang X, Ding X, Bin P, Zhu G. The vertical transmission of *Salmonella enteritidis* in a one-health context. One Health. 2023;**16**:100469. DOI: 10.1016/j.onehlt.2022.100469

[2] Dallman T, Ashton P, Schafer U, Jironkin A, Painset A, Shaaban S, et al. SnapperDB: A database solution for routine sequencing analysis of bacterial isolates. Bioinformatics. 2018;**34**:3028-3029. DOI: 10.1093/bioinformatics/bty212

[3] Afolami OI, Onifade AK. Antibiotic resistant *Salmonella* spp: Mechanism of drug resistance, gene variations and clinical implications. Asian Journal of Research in Medical and Pharmaceutical Sciences. 2018;**4**(4):1-6. DOI: 10.9734/AJRIMPS/2018/35958

[4] Falkow S. The evolution of pathogenicity in *E. coli*, *Shigella* and *Salmonella* spp. In: Neidhardt FC, Li J, Lin ECC, Low KB, Magasnik B, Reznikoff WS, Riloy M, Schaechter M, Umbarger HE, editors. *E. coli* and *Salmonella*: Cellular and Molecular Biology. Washington, DC: Am. Soci for Microbiol. Press; 1996. pp. 2723-2729

[5] Liebisch B, Schwarz SC. Evaluation and comparison of molecular techniques for epidemiological typing of *Salmonella enterica* subsp. *Enterica Serovar* Dublin. Journal of Clinical Microbiology. 1996;**34**:641-646

[6] Alenazy R. Antibiotic resistance in *Salmonella*: Targeting multidrug resistance by understanding efflux pumps, regulators and the inhibitors. Journal of King Saud University – Science. 2022;**34**:102275. DOI: 10.1016/j.jksus.2022.102275

[7] Podolak R, Enache E, Stone W, Black DG, Elliott PH. Sources and risk factors for contamination, survival, persistence, and heat resistance of *Salmonella* in low-moisture foods. Journal of Food Protection. 2010;**73**:1919-1936

[8] Ehuwa O, Jaiswal AK, Jaiswal S. *Salmonella*, food safety and food handling practices. Food. 2021;**10**:907. DOI: 10.3390/foods10050907

[9] Jacob M, World Health Organization. Safe Food Handling: A Training Guide for Managers in Food Service Establishments/Michael Jacob. World Health Organization; 1989. Available from: https://iris.who.int/handle/10665/36870

[10] WHO. WHO Guidelines on Use of Medically Important Antimicrobials in Food Producing Animals. Geneva: WHO; 2019. Available from: https://www.who.int/foodsafety/areas_work/antimicrobial-resistance/cia_guidelines/en/

[11] Yu H, Neal J, Dawson M, Madera JM. Implementation of behavior-based training can improve food service employees' handwashing frequencies, duration, and effectiveness. Cornell Hospitality Quarterly. 2018;**59**:70-77

[12] Stanaway JD, Parisi A, Sarkar K, Blacker BF, Reiner RC, Hay SI, et al. The global burden of non-typhoidal *Salmonella* invasive disease: A systematic analysis for the global burden of disease study 2017. The Lancet Infectious Diseases. 2019;**19**:1312-1324

[13] Kirk MD, Pires SM, Black RE, Caipo M, Crump JA, Devleesschauwer B, et al. World Health Organization estimates of the global and regional

disease burden of 22 foodborne bacterial, protozoal, and viral diseases, 2010: A data synthesis. PLoS Medicine. 2015;**12**:e1001921

[14] Simpson KM, Hill-Cawthorne GA, Ward MP, Mor SM. Diversity of *Salmonella* serotypes from humans, food, domestic animals and wildlife in New South Wales, Australia. BMC Infectious Diseases. 2018;**18**:1-11

[15] Forghani F, Sreenivasa MY, Jeon B. Editorial: One health approach to improve food safety. Frontiers in Microbiology. 2023;**14**:1269425. DOI: 10.3389/fmicb.2023.1269425

[16] Bronowski C, James CE, Winstanley C. Role of environmental survival in transmission of *Campylobacter jejuni*. FEMS Microbiology Letters. 2014;**356**:8-19

[17] Zinsstag J, Schelling E, Waltner-Toews D, Tanner M. From "one medicine" to "one health" and systemic approaches to health and well-being. Preventive Veterinary Medicine. 2011;**101**:148-156

[18] Sahin O, Morishita TY, Zhang Q. Campylobacter colonization in poultry: Sources of infection and modes of transmission. Animal Health Research Reviews. 2002;**3**:95-105

[19] Molina-Lopez RA, Valverdú N, Martin M, Mateu E, Obon E, Cerdà-Cuéllar M, et al. Wild raptors as carriers of antimicrobial-resistant *Salmonella* and *Campylobacter* strains. The Veterinary Record. 2011;**168**:565

[20] Aqeel M, Mirani AH, Ahmed Khoso P, Sahito J, Leghari R, Bhutto A, et al. A comprehensive study on one health strategy and public health effects of *Salmonella*. Journal of Bioresource Management. 2024;**11**(3):195-210

[21] WHO. Global Action Plan on Antimicrobial Resistance. Geneva, Switzerland: WHO Press, WHO Document Production Services; 2021. Available from: https://www.emro.who.int/health-topics/drug-resistance/global-action-plan.html

[22] Bandyopadhyay S, Samanta I. Antimicrobial resistance in agri-food chain and companion animals as a re-emerging menace in post-COVID epoch: Low-and middle-income countries perspective and mitigation strategies. Frontiers in Veterinary Science. 2020;7:620. DOI: 10.3389/fvets.2020.00620

[23] Belay WY, Getachew M, Tegegne BA, Teffera ZH, Dagne A, Zeleke TK, et al. Mechanism of antibacterial resistance, strategies and next-generation antimicrobials to contain antimicrobial resistance: A review. Frontiers in Pharmacology. 2024;**15**:1444781. DOI: 10.3389/fphar.2024.1444781

[24] Carrique-Mas JJ, Trung NV, Hoa NT, Mai HH, Thanh TH, Campbell JI, et al. Antimicrobial usage in chicken production in the Mekong Delta of Vietnam. Zoonoses and Public Health. 2015;**62**:70-78. DOI: 10.1111/zph. 12165

[25] Lloyd DH. Reservoirs of antimicrobial resistance in pet animals. Clinical Infectious Diseases. 2007;**45**:S148-S152. DOI: 10.1086/519254

[26] Cabello FC, Godfrey HP, Buschmann AH, Dölz HJ. Aquaculture as yet another environmental gateway to the development and globalisation of antimicrobial resistance. The Lancet Infectious Diseases. 2016;**16**:e127-e133. DOI: 10.1016/S1473-3099(16)00100-6

[27] Gunathilaka GU, Tahlan V, Mafiz AI, Polur M, Zhang Y. Phages in urban wastewater have the potential

to disseminate antibiotic resistance. International Journal of Antimicrobial Agents. 2017;**50**:678-683. DOI: 10.1016/j.ijantimicag.2017.08.013

[28] McNamara PJ, Levy SB. Triclosan: An instructive tale. Antimicrobial Agents and Chemotherapy. 2016;**60**:7015-7016. DOI: 10.1128/AAC.02105-16

[29] Kim M, Weigand MR, Oh S, Hatt JK, Krishnan R, Tezel U, et al. Widely used benzalkonium chloride disinfectants can promote antibiotic resistance. Applied and Environmental Microbiology. 2018;**84**:e01201-e01218. DOI: 10.1128/AEM.01 201-18

[30] Gulumbe BH, Adesola RO. Revisiting the blind spot of substandard and fake drugs as drivers of AMR in LMICs. Annals of Medicine and Surgery. 2023;**85**(2):122-123. DOI: 10.1097/MS9.00000 00000 000113

[31] Ahmad N, Joji RM, Shahid M. Evolution and implementation of one health to control the dissemination of antibiotic-resistant bacteria and resistance genes: A review. Frontiers in Cellular and Infection Microbiology. 2023;**12**:1065796. DOI: 10.3389/fcimb.2022.10657 96

[32] World Health Organization. Regional Office for South-East Asia. FAO-OIE-WHO One Health Approach to AMR Mitigation and Safer Food in the Asia-Pacific Region: 29-30 September 2021. World Health Organization. Regional Office for South-East Asia; 2022. Available from: https://iris.who.int/handle/10665/364712. License: CC BY-NC-SA 3.0 IGO

[33] Hibbard R, Mendelson M, Page SW, et al. Antimicrobial stewardship: A definition with a one health perspective. npj Antimicrobials and Resistance. 2024;**2**:15. DOI: 10.1038/s44259-024-00031-w

[34] Alhassan MY, Kabara MK, Ahmad AA, Abdulsalam J, Habib HI. Revisiting antibiotic stewardship: Veterinary contributions to combating antimicrobial resistance globally. Bulletin of the National Research Centre. 2025;**49**:25. DOI: 10.1186/s42269-025-01317-3

[35] Antimicrobial Resistance Collaborators. Global burden of bacterial antimicrobial resistance 1990-2021: A systematic analysis with forecasts to 2050. The Lancet. 2024;**404**(10459):1199-1226

[36] Velazquez-Meza ME, Galarde-López M, Carrillo-Quiróz B, Alpuche-Aranda CM. Antimicrobial resistance: One health approach. Veterinary World. 2022;**15**(3):743-749. DOI: 10.14202/vetworld.2022.743-749

[37] World Health Organization, Food and Agriculture Organization of the United Nations, United Nations Environment Programme & World Organisation for Animal Health. A One Health Priority Research Agenda for Antimicrobial Resistance. World Health Organization; 2023. Available from: https://iris.who.int/handle/10665/370279. License: CC BY-NC-SA 3.0 IGO

[38] World Health Organization. Prioritization of Pathogens to Guide Discovery, Research and Development of New Antibiotics for Drug-Resistant Bacterial Infections, Including Tuberculosis. World Health Organization; 2017. Available from: https://iris.who.int/handle/10665/311820. License: CC BY-NC-SA 3.0 IGO

[39] Bo L, Sun H, Li Y-D, Zhu J, Wurpel JND, Lin H, et al. Combating antimicrobial resistance: The silent war. Frontiers in Pharmacology.

2024;**15**:1347750. DOI: 10.3389/fphar.2024.1347750

[40] Uddin TM, Chakraborty AJ, Khusro A, Zidan BMRM, Mitra S, Emran TB, et al. Antibiotic resistance in microbes: History, mechanisms, therapeutic strategies and future prospects. Journal of Infection and Public Health. 2021;**14**:1750-1766. DOI: 10.1016/j.jiph.2021.10.020

[41] Yuce A. Mechanisms of acquiring resistance to antimicrobial drugs. Klimik Magazine. 2001;**14**(2):41-46

[42] D'Aquila P, De Rango F, Paparazzo E, Passarino G, Bellizzi D. Epigenetic-based regulation of transcriptome in *Escherichia coli* adaptive antibiotic resistance. Microbiology Spectrum. 2023;**11**:e0458322. DOI: 10.1128/spectrum.04583-22

[43] Lazar V, Oprea E, Ditu LM. Resistance, tolerance, virulence and bacterial pathogen fitness-current state and envisioned solutions for the near future. Pathogens. 2023;**12**:746. DOI: 10.3390/pathogens12050746

[44] Jawetz E, Melnick JL, Adelberg EA. Medical microbiology. East Norwalk, CT: Appleton and Lange; 1995. pp. 137-167

[45] Manchanda V, Sanchaita S, Singh NP. Multidrug resistant acinetobacter. Journal of Global Infectious Diseases. 2010;**2**:291-304. DOI: 10.4103/0974-777X.68538

[46] Gomez-Laguna J, Hernandez M, Creus E, Echeita A, Otal J. Prevalence and antimicrobial susceptibility of Salmonella infections in free-range pigs. The Veterinary Journal. 2010;**2**(5):18-24. DOI: 10.1016/j.tvji.2010.09.009

[47] Abdi SN, Ghotaslou R, Ganbarov K, Mobed A, Tanomand A, Yousefi M, et al. *Acinetobacter baumannii* efflux pumps and antibiotic resistance. Infection and Drug Resistance. 2020;**13**:423-434. DOI: 10.2147/IDR.S228089

[48] Crofts TS, Gasparrini AJ, Dantas G. Next-generation approaches to understand and combat the antibiotic resistome. Nature Reviews. Microbiology. 2017;**15**:422-434. DOI: 10.1038/nrmicro.2017.28

[49] Reygaert WC. An overview of the antimicrobial resistance mechanisms of bacteria. AIMS Microbiology. 2018;**4**(3):482-501. DOI: 10.3934/microbiol.2018.3.482

[50] Abdus Salam M, Al-Amin MY, Salam MT, Pawar JS, Akhter N, Rabaan AA, et al. Antimicrobial resistance: A growing serious threat for global public health. Healthcare. 2023;**11**:1946. DOI: 10.3390/healthcare11131946

[51] Blair JM, Webber MA, Baylay AJ, Ogbolu DO, Piddock LJ. Molecular mechanisms of antibiotic resistance. Nature Reviews. Microbiology. 2015;**13**:42-51. DOI: 10.1038/nrmicro3380

[52] Schaenzer AJ, Wright GD. Antibiotic resistance by enzymatic modification of antibiotic targets. Trends in Molecular Medicine. 2020;**26**(8):768-782. DOI: 10.1016/j.molmed.2020.05.001

[53] Ashley RE, Dittmore A, McPherson SA, Turnbough CL Jr, Neuman KC, Osheroff N. Activities of gyrase and topoisomerase IV on positively supercoiled DNA. Nucleic Acids Research. 2017;**45**:9611-9624. DOI: 10.1093/nar/gkx649

[54] Saha M, Sarkar A. Review on multiple facets of drug resistance: A rising challenge in the 21st century. Journal of Xenobiotics. 2021;**11**:197-214. DOI: 10.3390/jox11040013

[55] Eliopoulos GM, Huovinen P. Resistance to trimethoprim-sulfamethoxazole. Clinical Infectious Diseases. 2001;**32**(11):1608-1614. DOI: 10.1086/320532

[56] Reynolds D, Burnham JP, Guillamet CV, McCabe M, Yuenger V, Betthauser K, et al. The threat of multidrug-resistant/extensively drug-resistant gram-negative respiratory infections: Another pandemic. European Respiratory Review. 2022;**31**(166):1-20. DOI: 10.1183/16000617.0068-2022

[57] Baran A, Kwiatkowska A, Potocki L. Antibiotics and bacterial resistance-A short story of an endless arms race. International Journal of Molecular Sciences. 2023;**24**:5777. DOI: 10.3390/ijms24065777

[58] Fernández L, Hancock REW. Adaptive and mutational resistance: Role of porins and efflux pumps in drug resistance. Clinical Microbiology Reviews. 2012;**m25**(4):661-681. DOI: 10.1128/CMR.00043-12

[59] Choi U, Lee CR. Distinct roles of outer membrane porins in antibiotic resistance and membrane integrity in *Escherichia coli*. Frontiers in Microbiology. 2019;**10**:953. DOI: 10.3389/fmicb.2019.00953

[60] Palazzotti D, Felicetti T, Sabatini S, Moro S, Barreca ML, Sturlese M, et al. Fighting antimicrobial resistance: Insights on how the *Staphylococcus aureus* NorA efflux pump recognizes 2-phenylquinoline inhibitors by supervised molecular dynamics (SuMD) and molecular docking simulations. Journal of Chemical Information and Modeling. 2023;**63**:4875-4887. DOI: 10.1021/acs.jcim.3c00516

[61] Colclough AL, Alav I, Whittle EE, Pugh HL, Darby EM, Legood SW, et al. RND efflux pumps in Gram-negative bacteria; regulation, structure and role in antibiotic resistance. Future Microbiology. 2020;**15**:143-157. DOI: 10.2217/fmb-2019-0235

[62] Ragueh AA, Aboubaker MH, Mohamed SI, Rolain JM, Diene SM. Emergence of carbapenem-resistant gram-negative isolates in hospital settings in Djibouti. Antibiotics (Basel, Switzerland). 2023;**12**:1132. DOI: 10.3390/antibiotics12071132

[63] Beheshti M, Ardebili A, Beheshti F, Lari AR, Siyadatpanah A, Pournajaf A, et al. Tetracycline resistance mediated by tet efflux pumps in clinical isolates of *Acinetobacter baumannii*. Revista do Instituto de Medicina Tropical de São Paulo. 2020;**62**:e88. DOI: 10.1590/S1678-9946202062088

[64] Mingeot-Leclercq M, Decout J. Bacterial lipid membranes as promising targets to fight antimicrobial resistance, molecular foundations and illustration through the renewal of aminoglycoside antibiotics and emergence of amphiphilic aminoglycosides. MedChemComm. 2016;**7**:586-611. DOI: 10.1039/c5md00503e

[65] Diene SM, Pontarotti P, Azza S, Armstrong N, Pinault L, Chabriere E, et al. Origin, diversity, and multiple roles of enzymes with metallo-β-lactamase fold from different organisms. Cells. 2023;**12**:1752. DOI: 10.3390/cells12131752

[66] Tamma PDA, Samuel L, Bonomo RA, Mathers AJ, van Duin D, Clancy CJ. Infectious Diseases Society of America antimicrobial resistant treatment guidance: Gram-negative bacterial infections. A focus on extended-spectrum β-lactamase producing *Enterobacterales* (ESBL-E), carbapenem-resistant *Enterobacterales* (CRE), and *Pseudomonas aeruginosa* with

difficult-to-treat resistance (DTR-*P. Aeruginosa*). Infectious disease Society of America Practice Guidelines. Clinical Infectious Diseases. 2020;**72**:169-e183. DOI: 10.1093/cid/ciaa1478

[67] Queenan AM, Bush K. Carbapenemases: The versatile beta-lactamases. Clinical Microbiology Reviews. 2007;**20**:440-458. DOI: 10.1128/CMR.00001-07

[68] CDC. Antibiotic Resistance Threats in the United States, 2019. Atlanta, GA: U.S. Department of Health and Human Services, CDC; 2019

[69] Strateva T, Yordanov D. Pseudomonas aeruginosa - A phenomenon of bacterial resistance. Journal of Medical Microbiology. 2009;**58**:1133-1148. DOI: 10.1099/jmm.0.009142-0

[70] Jannat H, Shamsuzzaman SM, Faisal MA. Identification of genes encoding aminoglycoside modifying enzymes among clinical isolates of *Proteus* species at a tertiary care hospital in Dhaka, Bangladesh. Mymensingh Medical Journal : MMJ. 2022;**31**:289-294

[71] Anné J, Economou A, Bernaerts K. Protein secretion in gram-positive bacteria: From multiple pathways to biotechnology. In: Protein and Sugar Export and Assembly in Gram-Positive Bacteria. Cham, Switzerland: Springer; 2017. pp. 267-308

[72] Villageliu DN, Samuelson DR. The role of bacterial membrane vesicles in human health and disease. Frontiers in Microbiology. 2022;**13**:828704

[73] Magaña G, Harvey C, Taggart CC, Rodgers AM. Bacterial outer membrane vesicles: Role in pathogenesis and host-cell interactions. Antibiotics. 2024;**13**:32. DOI: 10.3390/antibiotics13010032

[74] Dhital S, Deo P, Bharathwaj M, Horan K, Nickson J, Azad M, et al. Neisseria gonorrhoeae-derived outer membrane vesicles package beta-lactamases to promote antibiotic resistance. Microlife. 2022;**3**:uqac013. Epub 2023/05/24. DOI: 10.1093/femsml/uqac013

[75] Huang W, Meng L, Chen Y, Dong Z, Peng Q. Bacterial outer membrane vesicles as potential biological nanomaterials for antibacterial therapy. Acta Biomaterialia. 2022;**140**:102-115

[76] Jiang B, Lai Y, Xiao W, Zhong T, Liu F, Gong J, et al. Microbial extracellular vesicles contribute to antimicrobial resistance. PLoS Pathogens. 2024;**20**(5):e1012143. DOI: 10.1371/journal.ppat.1012143

[77] May KL, Grabowicz M. The bacterial outer membrane is an evolving antibiotic barrier. Proceedings of the National Academy of Sciences of the United States of America. 2018;**115**(36):8852-8854. Epub 2018/08/25. DOI: 10.1073/pnas.1812779115

[78] Dhital S, Deo P, Bharathwaj M, Horan K, Nickson J, Azad M, et al. Neisseria gonorrhoeae-derived outer membrane vesicles package β-lactamases to promote antibiotic resistance. Microlife. 2022;**3**:uqac013

[79] Lopez C, Prunotto A, Bahr G, Bonomo RA, Gonzalez LJ, Dal Peraro M, et al. Specific protein-membrane interactions promote packaging of metallo-β-lactamases into outer membrane vesicles. Antimicrobial Agents and Chemotherapy. 2021;**65**(10):1-8. DOI: 10.1128/AAC.00507-21

[80] Toyofuku M, Schild S, Kaparakis-Liaskos M, Eberl L. Composition and functions of bacterial membrane vesicles. Nature Reviews. Microbiology.

2023;**21**(7):415-430. Epub 2023/03/19. DOI: 10.1038/s41579-023-00875-5

[81] Muñoz-Echeverri LM, Benavides-López S, Geiger O, Trujillo-Roldán MA, Valdez-Cruz NA. Bacterial extracellular vesicles: Biotechnological perspective for enhanced productivity. World Journal of Microbiology and Biotechnology. 2024;**40**:174

[82] Ciobanasu C. Bacterial extracellular vesicles and antimicrobial peptides: A synergistic approach to overcome antimicrobial resistance. MDPI Antibiotics. 2025;**14**:414. DOI: 10.3390/antibiotics14040414

[83] Rosenberg SM. Evolving responsively: Adaptive mutation. Nature Reviews Genetics. 2001;**2**:504-515

[84] Krašovec R, Jerman I. Bacterial multicellularity as a possible source of antibiotic resistance. Medical Hypotheses. 2003;**60**(4):484-488. DOI: 10.1016/S0306-9877(02)00394-8

[85] Foster PL. Adaptive mutation: Implications for evolution. BioEssays. 2000;**22**:1067-1074

[86] Higgins NP. Death and transfiguration among bacteria. Trends in Biochemical Sciences. 1992;**17**:207-211. DOI: 10.3390/antibiotics14040414

[87] Stewart PS, Costerton JW. Antibiotic resistance of bacteria in biofilms. Lancet. 2001;**358**:135-138

[88] Harshey RM, Toguchi A. Spinning tails: Homologies among bacterial flagellar systems. Trends in Microbiology. 1996;**4**:226-231

[89] Moens S, Vanderleyden J. Functions of bacterial flagella. Critical Reviews in Microbiology. 1996;**22**:67-100

[90] Romling U, Rohde M. Flagella modulate the multicellular behavior of *Salmonella typhimurium* on the community level. FEMS Microbiology Letters. 1999;**180**:91-102

[91] Romling U, Sierralta WD, Eriksson K, Normark S. Multicellular and aggregative behavior of *Salmonella typhimurium* strains is controlled by mutations in the agfD promoter. Molecular Microbiology. 1998;**28**:249-264

[92] Dutt Y, Dhiman R, Singh T, Vibhuti A, Gupta A, Pandey RP, et al. The association between biofilm formation and antimicrobial resistance with possible ingenious bio-remedial approaches. Antibiotics. 2022;**11**:930. DOI: 10.3390/antibiotics11070930

[93] Rutherford ST, Bassler BL. Bacterial quorum sensing: Its role in virulence and possibilities for its control. Cold Spring Harbor Perspectives in Medicine. 2012;**2**(11):a012427. DOI: 10.1101/cshperspect.a012427

[94] Britto CD, John J, Verghese VP, Pollard AJ. A systematic review of antimicrobial resistance of typhoidal *Salmonella* in India. The Indian Journal of Medical Research. 2019;**149**(2):151-163. DOI: 10.4103/ijmr.IJMR_830_18

[95] Britto CD et al. Persistent circulation of a fuoroquinolone-resistant *Salmonella enterica* Typhi clone in the Indian subcontinent. The Journal of Antimicrobial Chemotherapy. 2020;**75**(2):337-341. DOI: 10.1093/jac/dkz4935

[96] Katiyar A, Sharm P, Dahiya S, Singh H, Kapil A, Kaur P. Genomic profiling of antimicrobial resistance genes in clinical isolates of *Salmonella* Typhi from patients infected with typhoid fever in India. Scientific

Reports. 2020;**10**:8299. DOI: 10.1038/s41598-020-64934-0

[97] Mąka Ł, Popowska M. Antimicrobial resistance of *Salmonella* spp. isolated from food. Roczniki Państwowego Zakładu Higieny. 2016;**67**(4):343-358

[98] Ghaly TM, Gillings MR. New perspectives on mobile genetic elements: A paradigm shift for managing the antibiotic resistance crisis. Philosophical Transactions of the Royal Society of London. Series B, Biological Sciences. 2022;**377**:20200462. DOI: 10.1098/rstb.2020.0462

[99] Liu H, Zheng L, Fan H, Pang J. Genomic analysis of antibiotic resistance genes and mobile genetic elements in eight strains of nontyphoid *Salmonella*. mSystems. 2024;**9**(9):e0058624. DOI: 10.1128/msystems.00586-24

[100] Tokuda M, Shintani M. Microbial evolution through horizontal gene transfer by mobile genetic elements. Microbial Biotechnology. 2024;**17**:e14408. DOI: 10.1111/1751-7915.14408

[101] Aylward FO, Moniruzzaman M. Viral complexity. Biomolecules. 2022;**12**:1061

[102] Dion MB, Oechslin F, Moineau S. Phage diversity, genomics and phylogeny. Nature Reviews. Microbiology. 2020;**18**:125-138

[103] Botelho J. Defense systems are pervasive across chromosomally integrated mobile genetic elements and are inversely correlated to virulence and antimicrobial resistance. Nucleic Acids Research. 2023;**51**:4385-4397

[104] Delavat F, Miyazaki R, Carraro N, Pradervand N, van der Meer JR. The hidden life of integrative and conjugative elements. FEMS Microbiology Reviews. 2017;**41**:512-537

[105] Liu M, Li X, Xie Y, Bi D, Sun J, Li J, et al. ICEberg 2.0: An updated database of bacterial integrative and conjugative elements. Nucleic Acids Research. 2019;**47**:D660-D665

[106] Mahillon J, Chandler M. Insertion sequences. Microbiology and Molecular Biology Reviews. 1998;**62**:725-774

[107] Fonseca ÉL, Vicente AC. Integron functionality and genome innovation: An update on the subtle and smart strategy of integrase and gene cassette expression regulation. Microorganisms. 2022;**10**:224

[108] Deng Y, Bao X, Ji L, Chen L, Liu J, Miao J, et al. Resistance integrons: Class 1, 2 and 3 integrons. Annals of Clinical Microbiology and Antimicrobials. 2015;**14**:45

[109] Gillings MR. Class 1 integrons as invasive species. Current Opinion in Microbiology. 2017;**38**:10-15

[110] Brochet M, Couve E, Glaser P, Guedon G, Payot S. Integrative conjugative elements and related elements are major contributors to the genome diversity of *Streptococcus agalactiae*. Journal of Bacteriology. 2008;**190**:6913-6917. DOI: 10.1128/JB.00824-08

[111] Hall RM. *Salmonella* genomic islands and antibiotic resistance in *Salmonella enterica*. Future Microbiology. 2010;**5**:1525-1538. DOI: 10.2217/fmb.10.122

[112] Palmer KL, Kos VN, Gilmore MS. Horizontal gene transfer and the genomics of *Enterococcal* antibiotic resistance. Current Opinion in Microbiology. 2010;**13**:632-639. DOI: 10.1016/j.mib.2010.08.004

[113] Winter M, Buckling A, Harms K, Johnsen PJ, Vos M. Antimicrobial resistance acquisition via natural transformation: Context is everything. Current Opinion in Microbiology. 2021;**64**:133-138. DOI: 10.1016/j.mib.2021.09.009

[114] Sikorski J, Teschner N, Wackernagel W. Highly different levels of natural transformation are associated with genomic subgroups within a local population of *Pseudomonas stutzeri* from soil. Applied and Environmental Microbiology. 2002;**68**:865-873. DOI: 10.1128/aem.68.2.865-873.2002